Sudden Cardiac Death in the Young and Athletes

Gaetano Thiene
Domenico Corrado
Cristina Basso

Sudden Cardiac Death in the Young and Athletes

Text Atlas of Pathology and Clinical Correlates

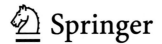 Springer

Gaetano Thiene
Cardiovascular Pathology
Department of Cardiac,
Thoracic and Vascular Sciences,
University of Padua,
Padova, Italy

Domenico Corrado
Cardiology
Department of Cardiac,
Thoracic and Vascular Sciences
University of Padua,
Padova, Italy

Cristina Basso
Cardiovascular Pathology
Department of Cardiac,
Thoracic and Vascular Sciences
University of Padua,
Padova, Italy

ISBN 978-88-470-5775-3   ISBN 978-88-470-5776-0   (eBook)
DOI 10.1007/978-88-470-5776-0

Library of Congress Control Number: 2016931987

Springer Milan Heidelberg New York Dordrecht London

Printed on acid-free paper

Springer-Verlag Italia Srl. is part of Springer Science+Business Media (www.springer.com)

Dedicated to the late Professor Lino Rossi, our mentor

Foreword

Sudden, unexpected cardiac death in a child, adolescent, or young adult is a catastrophic event for family, friends, and community. It is even more painful when it occurs in an apparently healthy young person who seems well enough to participate in athletic events. The public looks to the medical profession for an explanation for these tragic occurrences, but, since fortunately, they are relatively uncommon, most physicians – even cardiologists – have little experience with them, and, moreover, they do not even know where to look for answers when the need arises.

This situation has changed with the publication of this Text Atlas. Gaetano Thiene, Domenico Corrado, and Cristina Basso, Professors of Cardiovascular Pathology and Cardiology at the University of Padua, have devoted years to the careful study of these cases and now share their unique experience. The underlying causes of the arrhythmias, which are usually responsible for the sudden deaths, include a variety of congenital, valvular, and coronary arterial malformations, as well as a growing number of specific genetic and acquired cardiomyopathies and conduction system disorders. The gross and microscopic characteristics of these lesions are illustrated magnificently, and the clinical context is briefly but thoughtfully described. Some specimens are accompanied by pre-mortem electrocardiograms.

The approaches that the modern pathologist should use when faced with the heart of a victim of sudden death is an important chapter that will be quite useful. The authors recognize that some potentially fatal diseases, such as the channelopathies and other molecular disorders, may be fatal without leaving gross or microscopic traces. However, their presence can be inferred from electrocardiograms, more specialized electrophysiologic studies, as well as genetic screening.

Professors Thiene, Corrado, and Basso should be congratulated and thanked for this important contribution. The University of Padua provided a superb environment for this work. This University has an especially rich tradition in cardiology, dating back to the Renaissance. It was at Padua, where William Harvey, the discoverer of the circulation, received his medical training and was inspired to conduct the experiments leading to his momentous discovery. The clinical-pathologic correlations which form the core of this Text Atlas are a tradition introduced by the authors' distinguished eighteenth-century predecessor, the great Giovanni Battista Morgagni. This Text Atlas has been enriched by the collaboration of pathologists and clinicians in the Veneto region of Italy who have provided important specimens. Another unique feature that has facilitated interest in this field is the national policy for mandatory electrocardiographic screening of all people who wish to engage in athletics.

This Text Atlas will be of inestimable value to cardiac pathologists but will be of great interest to clinical cardiologists as well.

Boston, MA, USA   *Eugene Braunwald*

Contents

In the shape of a Text–Atlas, this is an overview of the pathology of sudden death (SD) in the young and in the athletes, summing up the experience we gathered in the perspective study carried out in the Veneto Region, Northeast of Italy.

Like at the time of Giovanni Maria Lancisi at the beginning of 1700, when a series of victims, "who in even other respects are healthy and vigorous," occurred in Rome thus alarming the population and the religious authorities, our interest on the topic started in the early 1980s following the autopsy of young people who died unexpectedly, either at rest or during exercise. These tragic events were touching since, as the great Leonardo da Vinci said, there is no science without feeling.

Thanks to the collaboration of forensic and anatomic pathologists of the Veneto Region, we set up a network able to cover the dissection of nearly all the cases of SD in people aged ≤35 years, with all the heart specimens and autopsy reports forwarded to the University of Padua.

It became soon evident that the majority of SD could find an explanation in hidden cardiac defects, threatening the electrical more than the mechanical properties of the heart and thus accounting for an abrupt arrhythmic "hearthquake" by ventricular fibrillation with cardiac arrest.

The singularity and novelty of the study was the availability, in many cases, of previous clinical investigations, thanks to the sport pre-participation screening including ECG that had become mandatory in Italy in 1982.

The method of clinicopathological correlation, which is at the base of our investigation following the historical tradition of Giovanni Battista Morgagni (1682–1771) at the University of Padua, allowed to detect the existence and to reconsider the value of subtle, apparently benign ECG abnormalities. Afterward, these anomalies were taken into serious attention at the pre-participation screening for further clinical investigations up to the final diagnosis and the definitive disqualification from sport activity. This experience played a fundamental role for putting forward criteria for the diagnosis of cardiomyopathies, which are the major cause of SD in the young and athletes. Mandatory screening, employment of ECG, and awareness by sport medicine doctors of the existence of hidden diseases at risk and how to diagnose them all were the key issues of the impressive results on prevention of SD, achieved simply through a "lifesaving" non-eligibility to sport activity and inherent lifestyle.

Along with the last 30 years, exciting scientific advances have been accomplished by clarifying the pathophysiologic mechanisms of cardiac arrest in the setting of a substrate: fibrofatty replacement in arrhythmogenic right cardiomyopathy (AC), disarray and fibrous scars in hypertrophic cardiomyopathy (HCM), and transient ischemia with myocardial injury in coronary artery disease, all aggravated by cardiac overload and ventricular wall stretching during exercise.

A not negligible part of the diseases at risk was found to be heredofamilial, with genetic carriers potentially at risk. The discovery of gene disorders allowed to identify the precise defective protein, thus establishing that HCM is a disease of the contractile apparatus (sarcomeric disease); AC, a disease of cell junctions (desmosomal disease); dilated cardiomyopathy mostly a disease of the cytoskeleton (cytoskelopathy); and SD without substrate (previously called "idiopathic" ventricular fibrillation) often a disease of ion channel/receptors (channelopathies). Indeed, nearly 15–20 % of cases do not exhibit at autopsy any gross and histological alteration (SD with normal heart). The skill of the pathologist is not only to find but also to exclude a morphological substrate, as to suggest the possible existence of ion channel or calcium receptor abnormalities. In these circumstances, the traditional tools of morphological investigation find a barrier in interpreting the phenomenon and should be associated to molecular investigation through polymerase chain reaction and gene sequencing, in order to identify the precise gene mutation ("molecular autopsy"). The existence of an ECG, recorded during life, as well as the circumstances of death and clinical history, may be of great help to address the genetic analysis. The alteration in these diseases with normal heart (long and short QT, Brugada, catecholaminergic syndromes) resides in the "morphology" of the ECG, whether at rest or on effort.

The use of molecular investigation plays a fundamental role also in establishing the precise etiology of myocarditis associated with SD, by detecting the viral genomes, either DNA or RNA. This was proven to be affordable even in paraffin-embedded tissue, thus helping to explain cases "left behind" from the archives.

This pathological experience with clinical correlates was useful to stratify the risk of these morbid entities, not only supporting the strategy of sport disqualification for those affected but also for therapy, particularly the employment of implantable cardioverter defibrillator (ICD), which revealed to be a "miraculous" tool in resuscitating from arrhythmic cardiac arrest.

Finally, and quite unexpectedly in the most optimistic perspectives of the 1980s when we started this venture, it was possible to recapitulate genetically determined cardiomyopathies in transgenic mice. It was really impressive, for instance, to realize how much it is possible to reproduce AC, similar to that occurring in humans, by introducing the homologous of the human gene defect in the mouse embryos' genome. This opens new avenues in the understanding of the basic molecular pathophysiology accounting for myocyte death and electrical instability.

Time will come when prevention of SD will be possible not only through symptomatic therapy by treating arrhythmias but also through a molecular therapy by understanding the pathobiological mechanisms. In other words, the aim will be not only to identify the subjects at risk, to disqualify them from exercise, and to treat with antiarrhythmic drugs, ablation, or ICD but also to cure the underlying biological defect. Molecular medicine is at the door.

The Authors

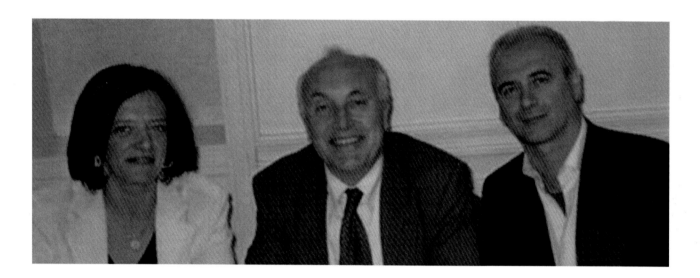

Acknowledgements This book was supported by the Registry of Cardio-Cerebro Vascular Pathology, Veneto Region, Venice, Italy; Strategic Research Project, TRANSAC, University of Padua, Italy; and Associazione Ricerche Cardiopatie Aritmiche-ARCA, Padua, Italy. The Authors thank Chiara Carturan, Marco Pizzigolotto, and all the staff of the Cardiovascular Pathology Unit at the University of Padua for their help and technical assistance.

2.1 Definition

SD is a natural phenomenon interrupting life instantaneously. The widely accepted definition is a death occurring unexpectedly, within 1 h from the onset of symptoms, in healthy even vigorous people or in people whose preexisting morbid conditions did not foresee such an abrupt outcome [1–18]. This temporal definition refers to witnessed SD, whereas it should be extended to 24 h for unwitnessed SD victims known to be alive and healthy one day prior to being found dead [3–7]. Since up to one third of SDs are unwitnessed, exclusion of these SDs would seriously bias a study by underrepresenting this quote. In nearly two third of cases, SD is the first cardiac event, whereas in one third it is predictable because the patient is at high risk. SD which takes place in the hospital has to be excluded, whereas that occurring in the emergency room is included.

SD may occur along with all the human life, even in prenatal time: up to 50 % of stillborn die suddenly in utero (sudden intrauterine unexplained death, i.e., SIUD, or stillbirth) [19]. Sudden unexpected infant death (SUID) affects infants with an incidence up to 1.5 % and may find an explanation at autopsy in unrecognized malformations, infections, or, not so rarely, following abuse [20]. Within SUID group, sudden infant death syndrome (SIDS) refers to SUID babies, 1–12 months old, found dead ("cot death"), in whom a cause is not discovered at autopsy. Nowadays, the incidence of SIDS varies from 0.3 to 1 % and is declining, following preventive measure with the supine position while sleeping.

2.2 Epidemiology

A recent systematic review of the publications dealing with the incidence of cardiac SD the United States clearly showed that very few studies have reported estimates from primary sources of data and that the stated definitions of cardiac SD and cardiac arrest are not standardized across the medical community [11].

In adolescents and young adults (<35 years) the incidence varies from 0.5 to 8/100,000/year in the reported epidemiological studies, and cardiomyopathies, myocarditis, premature coronary artery disease, congenital coronary artery anomalies, and channelopathies play a major causative role (Fig. 2.1) [2, 6–9, 21–23].

We carried out a prospective study in the Veneto Region, Northeast Italy, which holds a mean 4,379,900 overall population. Young population (12–35 years old) was 1,386,650 and young athletes 112,790, according to Italian Census Bureau & Sports Medicine database 1978–1999 [24]. The cumulative incidence of SD was 1/100,000/year. Among the non-athletic young people the incidence was 0.9/100,000/year, whereas in the athlete it was 2.3/100,000/year. Thus, the incidence of SD in athletes was 2.5-fold, clearly indicating that effort is at risk in people affected by hidden morbid entities, simply by unmasking them.

With age, the incidence of SD in general population is increasing, mostly due to coronary atherosclerosis but also to degenerative valve disease, like mitral valve prolapse and aortic stenosis [6–8]. However, coronary atherosclerosis may account for premature SD as early as at 25 years of age [25–28].

In the general population, SD may reach an incidence of 1 per 1000/year in the age interval 35–40 years, and 2 per 1000/year by 60 years [3, 8].

In the elderly (>60 years), SD is the mode of death in 25 % of cases, with an incidence up to 10–25 per 100/year in people affected by advanced ischemic heart disease. The incidence of SD increases dramatically as a function of advancing life, in parallel with the age-related increase of total coronary heart disease deaths. Overall, incidence of SD is 1 per 1000/year during the first year of life, 0.01 per 1000/year in adolescents and young adults (<35 years), 2 per 1000/year in adults, and 200 per 1000/year in the elderly.

There are two ages of peak of incidence of postnatal SD, one between 1 and 12 months (SUID and SIDS) and another over 45 years [8].

G. Thiene et al., *Sudden Cardiac Death in the Young and Athletes: Text Atlas of Pathology and Clinical Correlates*,
DOI 10.1007/978-88-470-5776-0_2

Nearly 50 % of all coronary heart disease deaths are sudden – unexpected and in two third SD is the first coronary event [6]. Half occurs out of the hospital or in emergency room and nearly 50 % of them have prior myocardial infarction. Diffuse obstructive coronary atherosclerosis and scars following previous myocardial infarction are the usual arrhythmogenic substrates found at autopsy. Coronary artery disease is the dominant cause of SD in the adult–elderly population (up to 80 %) [3–18].

The risk of coronary SD is 4–7 times greater in males compared to females in the young adult – middle-age population, because of the hormonal protection in females [3, 28, 29]. This does not exclude that classical coronary risk factors are predictor of events even in female (cigarette smoking, obesity, diabetes, hypertension, oral contraceptives) [6]. Smoking is the most important risk factor for SD even in women. Blood pressure levels and left ventricular hypertrophy have been also associated with a higher risk of SD [3].

Of course, the distribution of SD risk varies according to clinical and population profiles. The overall estimated incidence in the population is 0.1–0.2 % year, with total events of 300,000–350,000 deaths per year in the United States [10, 15] and nearly 50,000–60,000 deaths per year in Italy. Overall, event rates in Europe are similar to those in the United States [4], with significant geographic variations reported.

Obviously, the risk increases in higher-risk subgroups. For instance, the SD incidence is 1–2 %/year in people with coronary risk profile, 5 %/year in those with a prior coronary event, 15 %/year in those with congestive heart failure and ejection fraction (EF) <35 %, 25 %/year in cardiac arrest survivors. Combination of prior myocardial infarction, low EF, and ventricular tachycardia accounts for a risk of nearly 35 %/year [7] (Figs. 2.2 and 2.3).

These figures are now influenced by the benefit of drug (ß-blockers, amiodarone) and especially by implantable cardioverter defibrillator (ICD), according to evidence-based risk stratification.

However, nearly two third of SDs occur as the first clinical manifestation or, in the setting of known cardiac disease, in the absence of risk predictors. The cause is acute coronary thrombosis which precipitates upon nonobstructive, unstable atherosclerotic plaque, an event still unpredictable. Noteworthy, it is well known that 13–17 % of persons resuscitated from cardiac arrest develop an acute myocardial infarction [30, 31].

2.3 Pathophysiologic Mechanisms

Although the final pathway of SD is always cardiac arrest, the pathophysiologic mechanism may be cerebral, respiratory, and cardiovascular in origin when considering the primary loss of vital function [25–27, 32, 33].

Cerebral SD occurs as a consequence of cerebral hemorrhage, either intraparenchymal (usually hypertension) or subarachnoid (rupture of a congenital berry aneurysm). The latter is much more frequent in the young and may be considered the consequence of congenital dysplasia of the cerebral artery wall. The berry aneurysms are located throughout the cerebral circle of Willis, more frequently in the middle cerebral artery and in the anterior communicating artery (Fig. 2.4). Extensive hemispheric infarction after embolic occlusion of a carotid or cerebral artery may also account for SD. Brain injury occurs with cerebral edema, hernia of cerebellar tonsils into the occipital foramen, and injury of brain stem cardio-respiratory centers, with cardiac asystole as final mechanism of death.

Respiratory SD is the consequence of an abrupt obstruction of the airways, hindering lung ventilation and alveolar gas exchange. Suffocation and foreign body occlusion of upper airways (larynx, trachea, and bronchi) are accidental phenomena. Infectious inflammatory disease of the upper airways may lead to edema of the larynx with obstruction. However, the most common and frequent cause of respiratory SD in the young is allergic asthma, with bronchospasm and obstruction of the bronchi because of increased mucous secretion by bronchial glands (Fig. 2.5). The bronchial wall, with typical thickening of basal membrane and plugs in the bronchial lumen due to hypersecretion of the mucinous glands, appears infiltrated by eosinophils with amines release, accounting for bronchospasm. While in cerebral and cardiac SD loss of consciousness occurs immediately, during allergic asthma attack the patient is conscious and faces frightened the incoming death, becoming progressively cyanotic. Lack of blood oxygenation may contribute to slowdown of sinus node function and cardiac asystole.

SD in epilepsy (also known as sudden unexpected death in epilepsy, i.e., SUDEP) usually occurs during or immediately after an epileptic attack, through either cerebral or respiratory mechanism, insofar as the tonic–clonic seizure may jeopardize the brain stem respiratory centers or otherwise block the chest muscles with unpaired ventilation [34]. The risk of SD is 20 times higher than in the general population.

SD is cardiac (or cardiovascular) when the cardiac arrest is primarily due to a heart breakdown. Within a few minutes of cardiac arrest, irreversible cerebral damage occurs because of blood circulation stoppage. Cardiac arrest retains survival potential, thanks to prompt cardiopulmonary resuscitation maneuvers and defibrillators: if the subject survives from cardiac arrest, the term "aborted SD" is employed.

Cardiac arrest may be mechanical, when the heart function stops because of mechanical reasons. This is the case of pulmonary thromboembolism, when blood circulation is interrupted by the sudden occlusion of the pulmonary artery usually from a venous source (Fig. 2.6). In the young, it is often observed in women using estroprogestin drugs for therapeutic or contraceptive purpose, in obese people, and those with acquired or inherited hypercoagulable conditions, factor V Leiden being the most common [35].

Another circumstance of mechanical cardiovascular SD is hemopericardium with cardiac tamponade (Fig. 2.7). The amount of blood required to constrict the heart and impair diastolic ventricular filling is about 300–500 ml. Cause of hemopericardium may be cardiac rupture, complicating acute myocardial infarction; it usually occurs 2–4 days after the onset of myocardial infarcts, most often in the intensive coronary care unit (Fig. 2.8) and, as such, does not fit the definition of SD as an unpredictable event.

Instead, intrapericardial aortic rupture, due to aortic dissection, occurs suddenly and unexpectedly (whether due to hypertension, pregnancy, Marfan syndrome, or bicuspid aortic valve, with or without isthmic coarctation – see Chap. 7) (Fig. 2.9). In particular, while hypertension is the leading cause in the adult–elderly population, congenital or genetic diseases prevail in the young. Among the latter, Marfan syndrome is a genetic disorder, autosomal dominant, due to a mutation of fibrillin, a protein in the aortic wall tunica media connecting smooth muscle cells and elastic lamellae [36]. Besides extracardiac anomalies (lens luxation, arachnodactyly, laxity of the joints), it shows a peculiar cardiovascular involvement with progressive dilatation of the ascending aorta, accounting for aortic valve incompetence and eventually aortic dissection due to severe elastic disruption and medial necrosis in the tunica media [37]. A cut off of 5 cm aortic diameter is considered as the threshold for indication to surgery, to prevent the occurrence of aortic dissection and death.

Rupture of a concealed mycotic aneurysm into the pericardial sac may also account for cardiac tamponade (Fig. 2.10).

There are other circumstances which can abruptly interfere with blood circulation and vital organ perfusion. This is the case of acute hemorrhage, due to external rupture of either dissecting (usually thoracic) or atherosclerotic (either abdominal or thoracic) aortic aneurysm into the pleural cavity (which can host up to 2 liters of blood) or into the retroperitoneal space (Fig. 2.11), respectively. In both instances, which are almost exclusively observed in the adult–elderly population, hypovolemic shock occurs with cardiac asystole and death.

Acute mitral valve incompetence due to spontaneous rupture of chordae tendineae and mitral valve stenosis due to impingement of a huge left atrial myxoma are also exceptional causes of acute pulmonary edema and mechanical cardiac SD (Fig. 2.12).

SD may also occur in patients after heart valve replacement due to prosthetic valve dysfunction [38, 39]. Massive thrombosis with poppet block and embolization, as well as anticoagulation-related hemorrhage, are well-known complications. In cases of mechanical valve prostheses, abrupt detachment of annular suture anchorage, strut fracture, and tab fracture with valve leaflet escape (Fig. 2.13) are the main reported causes. In bioprostheses, sudden commissural tearing, either mechanical (Fig. 2.14) or related to calcification, is the equivalent of a strut fracture. These causes

usually account for acute pump failure and pulmonary edema.

Gastric or duodenal perforating ulcers may lead to a massive gastroduodenal hemorrhage and hypovolemic shock as well.

Shock may be septic in case of Waterhouse–Friderichsen syndrome, with bilateral adrenal hemorrhage, usually following meningococcal infection (Fig. 2.15). In this circumstance, shock is due to extreme dilatation of systemic microcirculation because of acute adrenal insufficiency. The overall size of blood circuit becomes exceedingly wider than the blood content, thus leading to severe hypotension, hypoxia, and eventually cardiac asystole.

However, the vast majority of primary cardiac SDs (more than 90 %) are arrhythmic ("electric cardiac SD") [3]. The pathophysiology may be asystole, due to sino-atrial or atrioventricular (AV) block; or, in the vast majority (>80 %), ventricular fibrillation (VF) (Fig. 2.16). Another mechanism is electromechanical dissociation, when electrical activity of the heart, still present, does not couple with contractility (pulseless electrical activity, PEA).

Also known as "heart delirium," VF is the most common final pathway of cardiac SD. There are several heart diseases which may complicate with VF and cardiac arrest: ischemic heart disease, cardiomyopathies, valve abnormalities, conduction system disorders, and ion channel diseases.

When recorded by ECG, often an early premature ventricular beat (R on T) is seen to trigger ventricular tachycardia (200–300 beats/min), which degenerates into ventricular flutter/VF (400–500 beats/min). The heart rate is too high and incompatible with an adequate diastolic filling/systolic stroke volume, thus leading to abrupt cessation of blood circulation and cerebral perfusion, loss of consciousness, and death in a few minutes.

VF is potentially reversible through an electric shock delivered by ICD or semiautomatic external defibrillator. They are "miraculous" lifesaving tools. Precise individual risk stratification should be put forward for indication of ICD. Automatic external defibrillators are going to be scattered in any public place and available for timely use, like fire extinguishers. Brain injury and death occur in a few minutes: survival declines by about 10 % per minute for patients in VF if prompt cardiopulmonary resuscitation manoeuvers and defibrillation are not applied [40, 41].

Overall, in our experience of SD in the young, nearly 90 % of SDs are primarily cardiovascular in origin, 5–7 % cerebral, and 3–5 % respiratory (Fig. 2.17). As far as cardiovascular SDs are concerned, they are mostly arrhythmic. However, adopting a larger time interval definition (24 h) from onset of symptoms to death, cardiac death among SD drops by nearly one third. In fact, the application of a 24-h definition of SD increases the fraction of all natural deaths falling into the "sudden" category but reduces the proportion of all SD that are due to cardiac causes, due to increased burden of cerebral death.

2.4   Image Gallery

Fig. 2.1 Association between the incidence of sudden death (SD) and age. The incidence of SD in adolescents and young adults (<35 years) varies from 0.5 to 8/100,000/year in the reported epidemiological studies. Note that SD is associated with various diseases throughout life. Cardiomyopathies, myocarditis, premature coronary artery disease, congenital coronary artery anomalies, and channelopathies play a major causative role in the young (From Myerburg and Vetter [8])

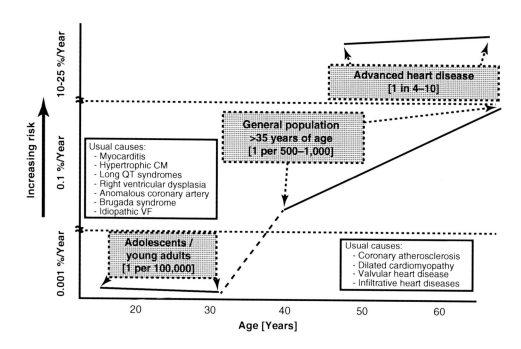

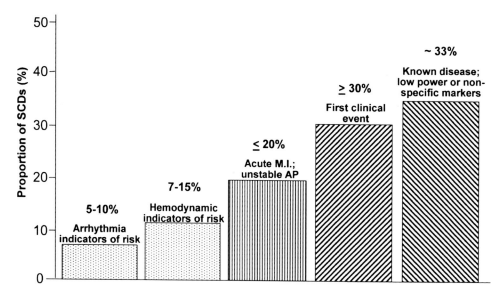

Fig. 2.2 The majority of out-of-hospital sudden cardiac death (SCD) occurs among either those patients in whom cardiac arrest is the first clinical expression of the underlying disease or those in whom disease is previously identified but classified as low risk. The so-called high-risk subgroups, such as post-myocardial infarction (MI) patients who manifest life-threatening arrhythmias and/or hemodynamic abnormalities and/or acute coronary syndromes, constitute a smaller proportion of the total SCD burden (From Myerburg and Castellanos [6])

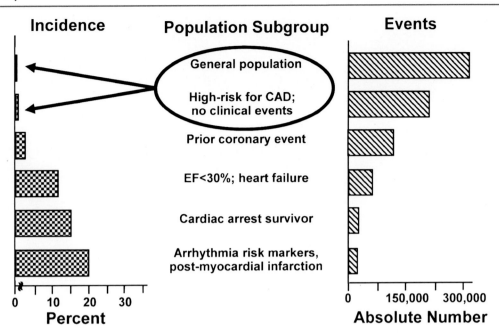

Fig. 2.3 Incidence and total population burden of sudden cardiac death. Incidence of event rates is compared with absolute numbers of events for the general population and for specific subgroups at risk. Note the inverse relationship between incidence and absolute numbers of events, indicating that a large portion of the total population burden emerges from subgroups with apparent no risk. *CAD* coronary artery disease, *EF* ejection fraction (From Myerburg and Junttila [9])

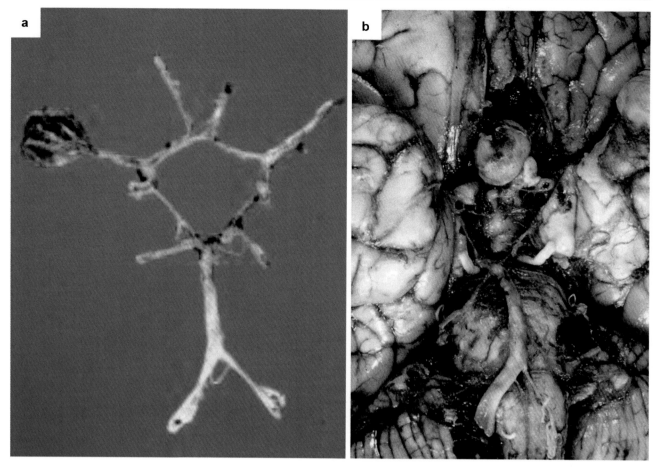

Fig. 2.4 Cerebral sudden death due to subarachnoid hemorrhage. Note the ruptured berry aneurysms of the middle right cerebral artery (**a**) and of the anterior communicating artery (**b**) of the Willis circle

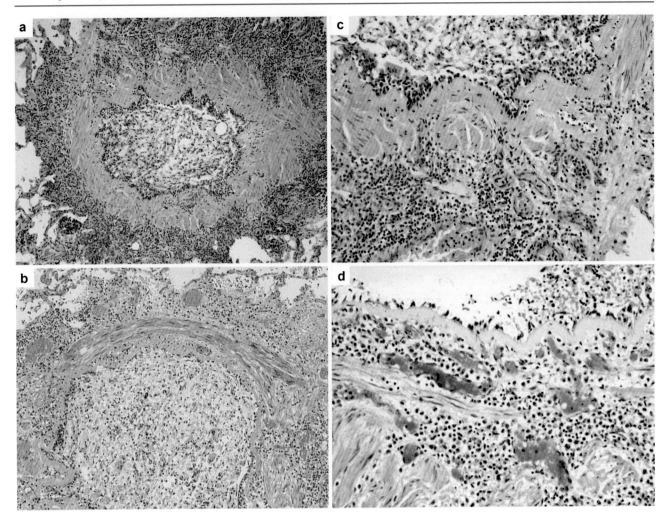

Fig. 2.5 Respiratory sudden death due to allergic asthma. Peripheral airway obstruction due to plugs in the bronchial lumen (**a**). Note the smooth muscle hypertrophy (**b**), the thickening of the bronchial basal membrane (**c**) and inflammatory infiltrate rich in eosinophils in the bronchial wall (**c, d**)

Fig. 2.6 Mechanical cardiovascular
sudden death. Saddle pulmonary
thromboembolism with abrupt blockage
of blood transit (**a**, **b**) extended from the
main trunk to proximal left and right
pulmonary arteries

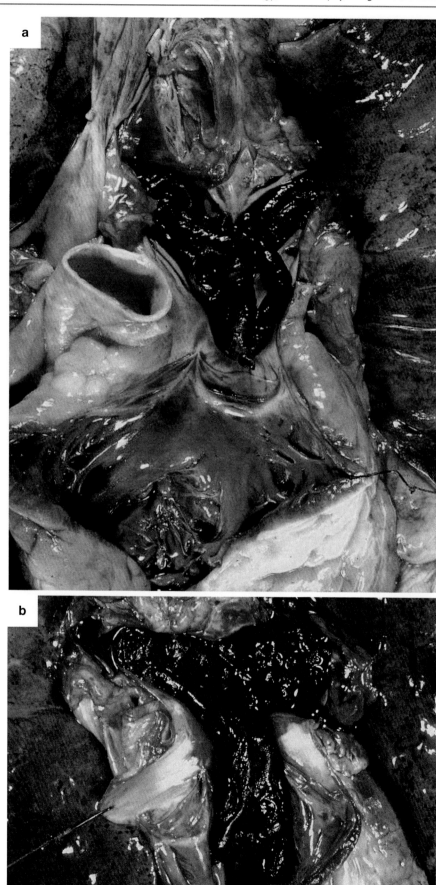

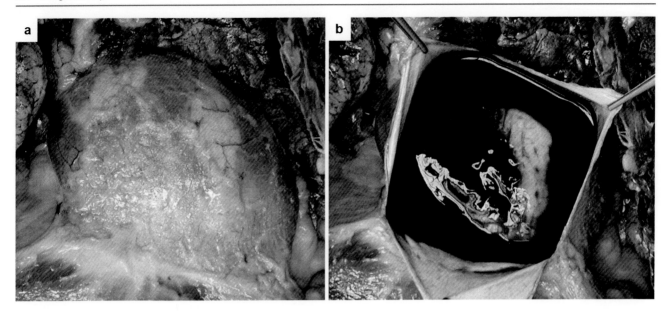

Fig. 2.7 Mechanical cardiovascular sudden death. Cardiac tamponade due to hemopericardium (**a**, **b**) impairs diastolic ventricular filling and cardiac output

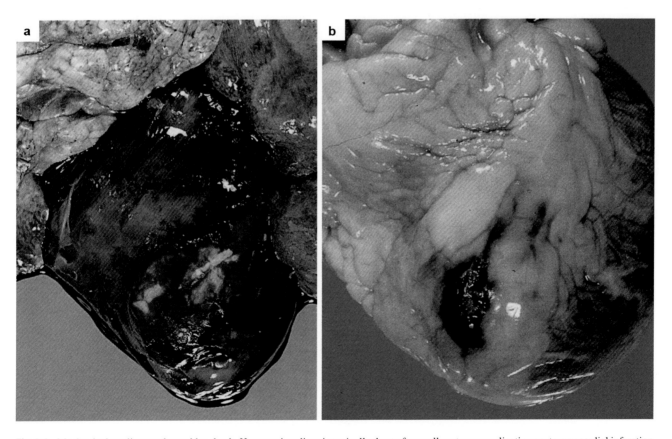

Fig. 2.8 Mechanical cardiovascular sudden death. Hemopericardium is typically due to free wall rupture complicating acute myocardial infarction (**a**, **b**)

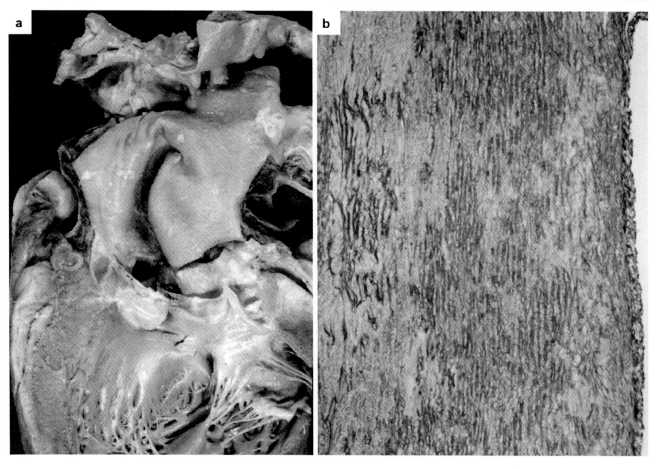

Fig. 2.9 Mechanical cardiovascular sudden death. Hemopericardium due to intrapericardial rupture of the ascending aorta in the setting of type A aortic dissection (**a**), with elastic fragmentation of the tunica media (**b**)

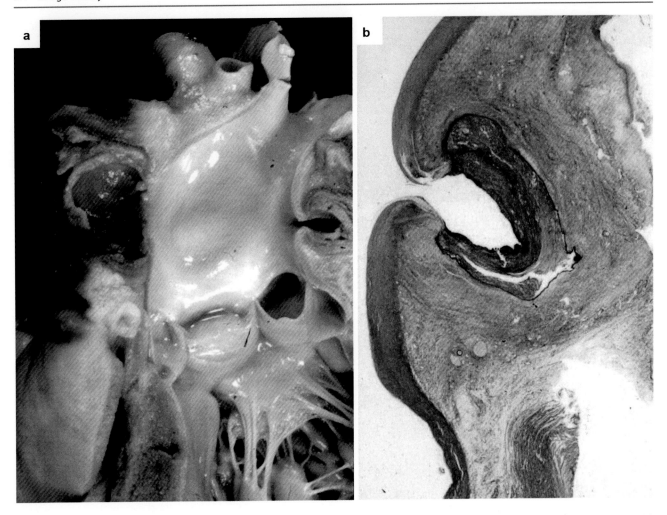

Fig. 2.10 Mechanical cardiovascular sudden death. Hemopericardium due to intrapericardial rupture of ascending aorta mycotic aneurysm (**a**) due to septic medial necrosis (**b**)

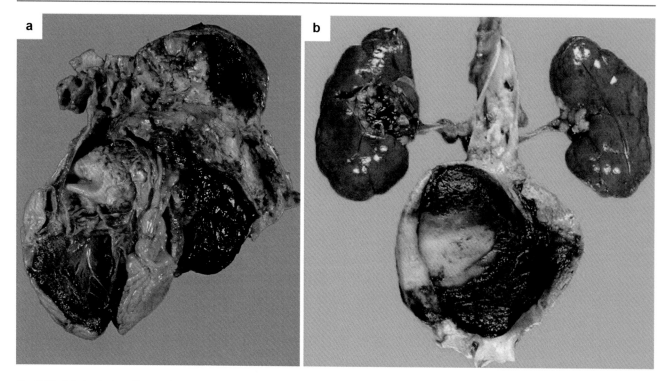

Fig. 2.11 Mechanical cardiovascular sudden death. Rupture of atherosclerotic aortic aneurysms into the left pleural cavity (**a**) and into peritoneal or retroperitoneal space (**b**), with acute hypovolemia and hemorrhagic shock

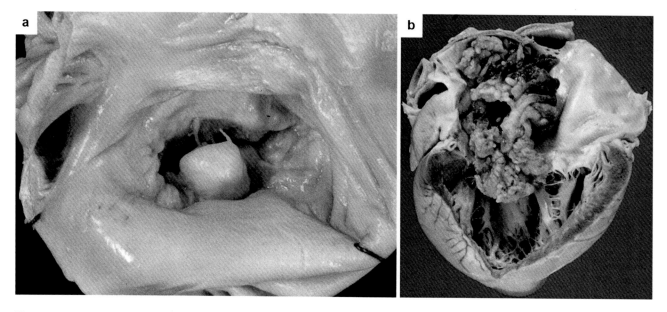

Fig. 2.12 Mechanical cardiovascular sudden death. Acute severe mitral incompetence (**a**) due to spontaneous rupture of chordae tendineae or mitral valve orifice occlusion (**b**) due to huge mobile atrial myxoma, with pulmonary edema

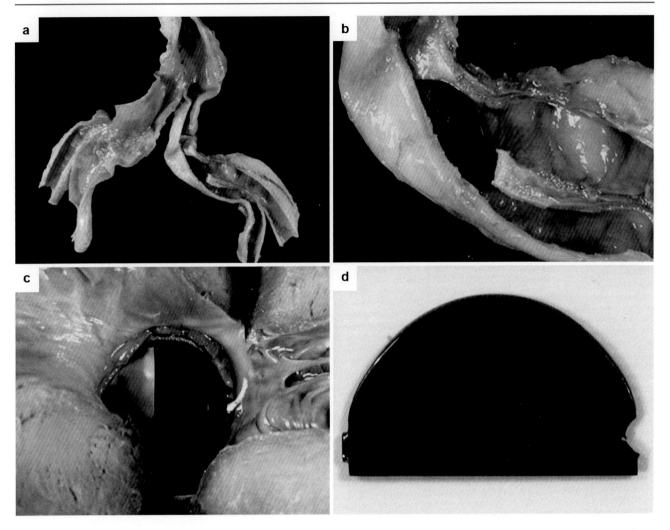

Fig. 2.13 Mechanical cardiovascular sudden death due to valve leaflet escape as a consequence of tab fracture in a patient with aortic valve replacement with a TRI-tech mechanical prosthesis. (**a**) Aortic Carrefour: the TRI-tech valve leaflet, escaped from the aortic position, is visible at the bifurcation of the left common iliac artery. (**b**) A close-up view of picture A. (**c**) In the aortic position, a leaflet of the TRI-tech valve is missing. (**d**) The missing leaflet, found in the left common iliac artery, with a tab asymmetry

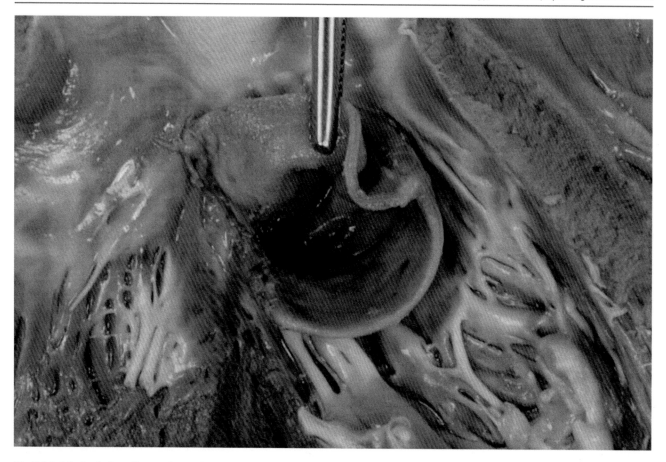

Fig. 2.14 Mechanical cardiovascular sudden death after mitral valve replacement with a unicusp pericardial bioprosthesis. An abrupt cuspal tear at one commissure led to severe mitral incompetence and pulmonary edema

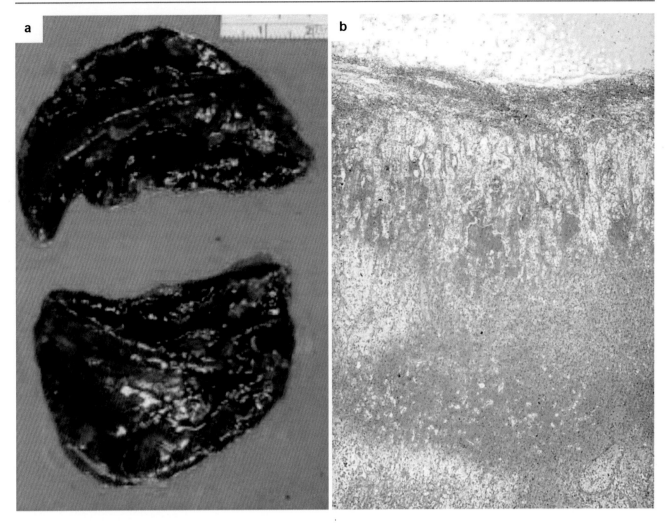

Fig. 2.15 Mechanical cardiovascular sudden death. Septic shock in Waterhouse–Friderichsen syndrome (also known as hemorrhagic adrenalitis or fulminant meningococcemia) with fall of blood pressure. Note the bleeding apoplexy of the adrenal glands with acute adrenal insufficiency, caused by severe bacterial infection (most commonly meningococcus). (**a**) gross appearance of hemorrhagic adrenal glands; (**b**) histology with evidence of hemorrhagic adrenalitis

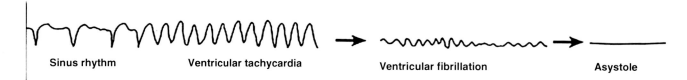

Fig. 2.16 Arrhythmic cardiac sudden death. Ventricular fibrillation, usually complicating ventricular tachycardia, is by far the most common pathophysiologic mechanism of sudden death

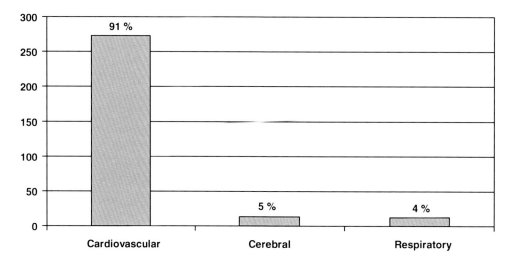

Fig. 2.17 Pathophysiologic mechanisms of sudden death in young people aged ≤35 years. The majority are cardiovascular in origin (91 %), followed by cerebral (5 %) and respiratory (4 %)

References

1. Goldstein S. The necessity of a uniform definition of sudden coronary death: witnessed death within 1 hour of the onset of acute symptoms. Am Heart J. 1982;103:156–9.

2. Myerburg RJ, Kessler KM, Castellanos A. Sudden cardiac death, Structure, function and time-dependence of risk. Circulation. 1992;85 Suppl 1:I2–10.

3. Zipes DP, Camm AJ, Borggrefe M, Buxton AE, Chaitman B, Fromer M, Gregoratos G, Klein G, Moss AJ, Myerburg RJ, Priori SG, Quinones MA, Roden DM, Silka MJ, Tracy C, Smith Jr SC, Jacobs AK, Adams CD, Antman EM, Anderson JL, Hunt SA, Halperin JL, Nishimura R, Ornato JP, Page RL, Riegel B, Blanc JJ, Budaj A, Dean V, Deckers JW, Despres C, Dickstein K, Lekakis J, McGregor K, Metra M, Morais J, Osterspey A, Tamargo JL, Zamorano JL, American College of Cardiology/American Heart Association Task Force, European Society of Cardiology Committee for Practice Guidelines, European Heart Rhythm Association; Heart Rhythm Society. ACC/AHA/ESC 2006 guidelines for management of patients with ventricular arrhythmias and the prevention of sudden cardiac death: a report of the ACC/AHA task force and the ESC committee for practice guidelines. Circulation. 2006;114:e385–484.

4. Priori SG, Aliot E, Blomstrom-Lundqvist C, Bossaert L, Breithardt G, Brugada P, Camm AJ, Cappato R, Cobbe SM, Di Mario C, Maron BJ, McKenna WJ, Pedersen AK, Ravens U, Schwartz PJ, Trusz-Gluza M, Vardas P, Wellens HJ, Zipes DP. Task force on sudden cardiac death of the European Society of Cardiology. Eur Heart J. 2001;22:1374–450.

5. Manolio TA, Furberg CD. Epidemiology of sudden cardiac death. In: Akhtar M, Myerburg RJ, Ruskin JN, editors. Sudden cardiac death. Malvern: William & Wilkins; 1994. p. 3–20.

6. Myerburg RJ, Castellanos A. Cardiac arrest and sudden cardiac death. In: Braunwald E, editor. Heart disease: a textbook of cardiovascular medicine. Philadelphia: WB Saunders; 2001. p. 890–931.

7. Myerburg RJ. Sudden cardiac death: exploring the limits of our knowledge. J Cardiovasc Electrophysiol. 2001;12:369–81.

8. Myerburg RJ, Vetter VL. Electrocardiograms should be included in preparticipation screening of athletes. Circulation. 2007;116:2616–26.

9. Myerburg RJ, Junttila MJ. Sudden cardiac death caused by coronary heart disease. Circulation. 2012;125:1043–52.

10. Deo R, Albert CM. Epidemiology and genetics of sudden cardiac death. Circulation. 2012;125:620–37.

11. Kong MH, Fonarow GC, Peterson ED, Curtis AB, Hernandez AF, Sanders GD, Thomas KL, Hayes DL, Al-Khatib SM. Systematic review of the incidence of sudden cardiac death in the United States. J Am Coll Cardiol. 2011;57:794–801.

12. Stecker EC, Reinier K, Marijon E, Narayanan K, Teodorescu C, Uy-Evanado A, Gunson K, Jui J, Chugh SS. Public health burden of sudden cardiac death in the United States. Circ Arrhythm Electrophysiol. 2014;7:212–7.

13. Goldberger JJ, Basu A, Boineau R, Buxton AE, Cain ME, Canty Jr JM, Chen PS, Chugh SS, Costantini O, Exner DV, Kadish AH, Lee B, Lloyd-Jones D, Moss AJ, Myerburg RJ, Olgin JE, Passman R, Stevenson WG, Tomaselli GF, Zareba W, Zipes DP, Zoloth L. Risk stratification for sudden cardiac death: a plan for the future. Circulation. 2014;129:516–26.

14. Chugh SS, Jui J, Gunson K, Stecker EC, John BT, Thompson B, Ilias N, Vickers C, Dogra V, Daya M, Kron J, Zheng ZJ, Mensah G, McAnulty J. Current burden of sudden cardiac death: multiple source surveillance versus retrospective death certificate-based review in a large U.S. community. J Am Coll Cardiol. 2004;44:1268–75.

15. Chugh SS, Reinier K, Teodorescu C, Evanado A, Kehr E, Al Samara M, Mariani R, Gunson K, Jui J. Epidemiology of sudden cardiac death: clinical and research implications. Prog Cardiovasc Dis. 2008;51:213–28.

16. Gillum RF. Sudden coronary death in the United States: 1980–1985. Circulation. 1989;79:756–65.

17. Zheng ZJ, Croft JB, Giles WH, Mensah GA. Sudden cardiac death in the United States, 1989 to 1998. Circulation. 2001;104:2158–63.

18. Becker LB, Smith DW, Rhodes KV. Incidence of cardiac arrest: a neglected factor in evaluating survival rates. Ann Emerg Med. 1993;22:86–91.

19. Stillbirth Collaborative Research Network Writing Group. Causes of death among stillbirths. JAMA. 2011;306:2459–68.

20. Kinney HC, Thach BT. The sudden infant death syndrome. N Engl J Med. 2009;361:795–805.

21. Silka MJ, Kron J, Walance CG, Cutler JE, McAnulty JH. Assessment and follow-up of pediatric survivors of sudden cardiac death. Circulation. 1990;82:341–9.

22. Driscoll DJ, Edwards WD. Sudden unexpected death in children and adolescents. J Am Coll Cardiol. 1985;5(6 Suppl):118B–21.

23. Shen WK, Edwards WD, Hammill SC, Bailey KR, Ballard DJ, Gersh BJ. Sudden unexpected nontraumatic death in 54 young adults: a 30-year population-based study. Am J Cardiol. 1995;76:148–52.

24. Corrado D, Basso C, Rizzoli G, Schiavon M, Thiene G. Does sports activity enhance the risk of sudden death in adolescents and young adults? J Am Coll Cardiol. 2003;42:1959–63.

25. Thiene G, Basso C, Corrado D. Cardiovascular causes of sudden death. In: Silver MD, Gotlieb AI, Schoen FJ, editors. Cardiovascular pathology. Philadelphia: Churchill Livingstone; 2001. p. 326–74.

26. Thiene G, Carturan E, Corrado D, Basso C. Prevention of sudden cardiac death in the young and in athletes: dream or reality? Cardiovasc Pathol. 2010;19:207–17.

27. Basso C, Calabrese F, Corrado D, Thiene G. Postmortem diagnosis in sudden cardiac death victims: macroscopic, microscopic and molecular findings. Cardiovasc Res. 2001;50:290–330.

28. Albert CM, Chae CU, Grodstein F, Rose LM, Rexrode KM, Ruskin JN, Stampfer MJ, Manson JE. Prospective study of sudden cardiac death among women in the United States. Circulation. 2003;107:2096–101.

29. Doyle JT, Kannel WB, McNamara PM, Quickenton P, Gordon T. Factors related to suddenness of death from coronary disease: combined Albany-Framingham studies. Am J Cardiol. 1976;37:1073–8.

30. Schaffer WA, Cobb LA. Recurrent ventricular fibrillation and modes of death in survivors of out-of-hospital ventricular fibrillation. N Engl J Med. 1975;293:259–62.

31. Baum RS, Alvarez 3rd H, Cobb LA. Survival after resuscitation from out-of-hospital ventricular fibrillation. Circulation. 1974;50:1231–5.

32. Roberts WC. Sudden cardiac death: definitions and causes. Am J Cardiol. 1986;57:1410–3.

33. Basso C, Burke M, Fornes P, Gallagher PJ, de Gouveia RH, Sheppard M, Thiene G, van der Wal A, Association for European Cardiovascular Pathology. Guidelines for autopsy investigation of sudden cardiac death. Virchows Arch. 2008;452:11–8.

34. Shorvon S, Tomson T. Sudden unexpected death in epilepsy. Lancet. 2011;378:2028–38.

35. Goldhaber SZ. Pulmonary embolism. Lancet. 2004;363:1295–305.

36. Loeys BL, Dietz HC, Braverman AC, Callewaert BL, De Backer J, Devereux RB, Hilhorst-Hofstee Y, Jondeau G, Faivre L, Milewicz DM, Pyeritz RE, Sponseller PD, Wordsworth P, De Paepe AM. The revised Ghent nosology for the Marfan syndrome. J Med Genet. 2010;47:476–85.

37. Chiu HH, Wu MH, Chen HC, Kao FY, Huang SK. Epidemiological profile of Marfan syndrome in a general population: a national database study. Mayo Clin Proc. 2014;89: 34–42.

38. Burke AP, Farb A, Sessums L, Virmani R. Causes of sudden cardiac death in patients with replacement valves: an autopsy study. J Heart Valve Dis. 1994;3:10–6.

39. Della Barbera M, Bottio T, Angelini A, Cresce GD, Montisci M, Gerosa G, Valente M, Thiene G. The pathology of TRI-Tech valve leaflet escape. J Heart Valve Dis. 2012;21:241–6.

40. Rea TD, Page RL. Community approaches to improve resuscitation after out-of-hospital sudden cardiac arrest. Circulation. 2010;121:1134–40.

41. Estes 3rd NA. Predicting and preventing sudden cardiac death. Circulation. 2011;124:651–6.

Sudden cardiac death (SCD) is mostly ascribable to coronary artery disease and is due to a large spectrum of both congenital and acquired morbid entities [1–3]. Premature coronary atherosclerosis is ranking first even in young age, with peculiar features of an accelerated proliferative phenomenon [2, 4].

3.1 Atherosclerotic Coronary Artery Disease

The disease and the mechanisms of cardiac arrest in the young are peculiar insofar as:

1. In contrast with SCD in the adult and elderly, thrombotic occlusion of a main subepicardial coronary artery is not the rule. Only 25–30 % of cases present with recent occlusive thrombosis [2, 4].
2. The phenomenon is mostly focal, consisting of a single vessel disease in contrast with the adult and elderly population where a diffuse, multivessel involvement is typically found (Fig. 3.1). The obstructive (>75 % lumen stenosis), usually eccentric, atherosclerotic plaque is often located in the proximal tract of the anterior descending branch of the left coronary artery [2, 4] (Fig. 3.2).
3. The culprit lesion rarely shows the classic features of vulnerable atherosclerotic plaque (necrotic core covered by a thin fibrous cap) [1, 5–8] (Figs. 3.3 and 3.4). It is mostly fibrocellular, due to recent smooth muscle cell growth indicating an accelerated proliferative phenomenon [2, 4, 9–15] (Figs. 3.1, 3.5, 3.6, and 3.7).
4. When thrombotic occlusion is observed, the thrombosis rarely precipitates as a consequence of plaque rupture or fissuring of the atherosclerotic plaque with thin fibrous cap [2, 4] (Figs. 3.8, 3.9, and 3.10). The thrombus is a mixture of platelets and fibrin entrapping red cells (Fig. 3.11). More frequently, endothelial erosion accounts for thrombogenicity [16, 17] (Figs. 3.12 and 3.13) and inflammation of the superficial layer of the intima ("endo-

thelitis") is often observed as a cause of endothelial cell detachment (Fig. 3.14). In the setting of endothelial erosion due to extensive T-lymphocytes and macrophage infiltration, molecular pathology investigation can help in detecting viral infection as a cause of coronary plaque instability precipitating thrombotic occlusion [18] (Fig. 3.15). The thrombosis may be occlusive or mural (Fig. 3.16). In both conditions, detachment of thrombus fragments may lead to embolism into the distal coronary small arteries (Fig. 3.17).

5. In the absence of an organic occlusion of a coronary artery, as in the case of a single obstructive atherosclerotic plaque, a transient ischemic attack, most probably due to vasospasm, has been demonstrated to occur just before cardiac arrest, with ST segment elevation on ECG like in Prinzmetal variant angina [12, 14, 19, 20] (Figs. 3.18 and 3.19). Reperfusion, following release of vasospasm, entails life-threatening electrical instability, because of massive calcium cellular inflow, due to damage of sarcolemma following transient myocardial ischemia.
6. Risk factors for accelerated atherosclerotic coronary artery disease leading to SCD in the young are not easily recognizable, due to the almost absent clinical information, including laboratory tests, in this apparently healthy population. Among the risk factors, cocaine and other drug addiction are well known particularly in young adults [21, 22]. Systematic toxicology investigation indicated that about 3 % of SCD are cocaine-related, and premature coronary artery atherosclerosis, with or without lumen thrombosis, is a frequent finding that may account for myocardial ischemia at risk of cardiac arrest in cocaine addicts [21] (Fig. 3.20). Small vessel disease is quite often associated with epicardial atherosclerotic coronary artery disease in this population (Fig. 3.21).
7. In our extensive experience of SCD in the young, an overt acute myocardial infarction was rarely observed, even at histology, and myocardial scar due to previous infarction was also quite rare (Fig. 3.22) [4], in contrast with the adult

© Springer-Verlag Milan 2016
G. Thiene et al., *Sudden Cardiac Death in the Young and Athletes: Text Atlas of Pathology and Clinical Correlates*,
DOI 10.1007/978-88-470-5776-0_3

elderly population [1, 23, 24] (Figs. 3.1 and 3.23). Because of the instantaneous death, it is impossible to predict whether these young people would have developed overt myocardial infarction, if resuscitated. Certainly, in case of fresh occlusive thrombosis, the occurrence of cardiac arrest due to ventricular fibrillation is most probably equivalent to that occurring within the first hour of myocardial infarction with out-of-the-hospital fatal outcome [25–28]. In case of transient coronary artery occlusion following vasospasm, it is also impossible to establish whether the constriction time would have been long enough to precipitate an acute myocardial infarction, either subendocardial or even transmural. It is well known that histological evidence of myocardial infarction is detectable not before 3–4 h from the time of coronary occlusion. It is highly probable that, like in experimental ligation of the descending coronary artery in the dog which immediately triggers ventricular fibrillation, transient ischemia due to vasospasm may be enough to threaten the regular electrical impulse transmission or favor ectopic ventricular tachycardia by triggered activity. A genetic predisposition to ventricular fibrillation has been suggested with a specific single nucleotide polymorphism in chromosome 21q21 [29]. A pathological substrate in the myocardium, consistent with a reentry mechanism for ventricular arrhythmias, is lacking in the absence of fibrous scars (Fig. 3.23) and the hypothesis that transient ischemia may precipitate an ion channel disorder cannot be ruled out.

Summing up, atherosclerotic SCD in the young is mostly due to a vasospastic transient coronary occlusion at the level of a single non-atheromatous obstructive plaque, located in the first tract of the left anterior descending branch (i.e., functional plaque instability in the form of vasospasm). When coronary artery occlusion is due to thrombosis, the latter occurs more frequently upon endothelial erosion rather than fibrous cap rupture. Gross and/or histological evidences of acute/chronic myocardial infarction are rare.

3.2 Non-atherosclerotic Coronary Artery Disease

One third of the cases of fatal coronary artery disease in the young are non-atherosclerotic and can be either acquired or congenital, with coronary artery anomalies being the most frequent form [30–32].

3.2.1 Embolism

Embolism may complicate cardiac disease of the left-sided heart with mural thrombosis (atrial fibrillation, dilated cardiomyopathy, acute and chronic myocardial infarction) and the coronary arterial tree may be the target [33] (Fig. 3.24). However, these conditions are extremely rare in the young and athletes. More frequently, a coronary embolism may occur in the presence of left atrial myxoma (Fig. 3.25) or endocardial fibroelastoma [34–36]. While in the setting of cardiac myxoma the embolism may be neoplastic because of the detachment of myxoid tissue from a villous and friable mass, in the setting of endocardial fibroelastoma the embolus is mostly thrombotic in nature because of stratification of fibrin over or within the fronds of the tumor, followed by detachment. In contrast with the villi of myxoma, the fronds of a papilloma present with a firm fibroelastic stalk, almost impossible to detach. However, tumor embolization cannot be excluded, since rare cases have been reported with distal embolism and histological evidence of neoplastic nature even in cases with endocardial fibroelastic papilloma. When the tumour grows upon a coronary aortic cusp, it may herniate into and occlude the coronary ostium, thus precipitating cardiac arrest [37]. Septic coronary embolism may occur in the setting of infective endocarditis and cause SCD, but of course this does not usually occur unexpectedly in a healthy subject [38] (Fig. 3.26).

3.2.2 Arteritis

Necrotizing noninfectious arteritis may involve the coronary arteries and account for coronary occlusion and SCD. This is the case of Kawasaki disease, which is featured by a peculiar involvement of the coronary arterial tree and characterized by a tendency to aneurysmal formation, because of tunica media inflammatory necrosis, and lumen thrombotic occlusion, leading to myocardial infarction and chronic ischemic heart disease [39–41] (Fig. 3.27).

Giant cell arteritis may also involve the coronary arteries [42, 43]. With specific reference in the young, this is the case of Takayasu's arteritis which usually affects young women and involves the aortic arch and brachiocephalic arteries with severe stenosis and subclavian "steal." The intrapericardial great arteries may be involved as well. When the ascending aorta is affected, the inflammation may be extended to the coronary ostia with lumen obstruction, so severe to precipitate myocardial ischemia and SCD (Fig. 3.28). In contrast of Kawasaki disease, it is not associated with aneurysm because of peri-adventitial fibrotic coating.

3.2.3 Dissection

It is a coronary disease typical of young–middle-aged women, frequently occurring in the peripartum period [44–47]. It is characterized by sudden lumen occlusion because of dissecting hematoma of the tunica media of the main subepicardial coronary arteries (Fig. 3.29), usually the left trunk and the descending coronary artery, but also the right coronary artery and other coronary branches. The hematoma pushes the intimal-inner-medial layers into and occludes the true lumen [44, 47] (Figs. 3.30 and 3.31). Sudden cardiac arrest is the frequent clinical presentation, as it is in coronary occlusion by thrombosis upon atherosclerotic plaque or by coronary embolism.

In contrast with the aorta, where dissection represents the most frequent form of acute aortic syndrome, SCD in coronary dissection is not "mechanical" due to external rupture with cardiac tamponade. On the opposite, it occurs through an acute myocardial ischemia with ventricular fibrillation. The pathogenesis of dissection is controversial. The "fragility" of the coronary tunica media is not comparable to that of the aorta. The coronary artery wall is muscular, the aortic one is elastic. Erdheim's cystic medial necrosis is rarely observed in coronary dissection. The only peculiar, frequently reported, histological feature is an eosinophilic inflammatory infiltrate in the outer tunica media and adventitia as to advance the hypothesis of an allergic arteritis [44, 48, 49] (Fig. 3.31). Its significance remains obscure since coronary dissection is not a typical finding in allergic syndromes and the eosinophilic infiltrate is mostly confined to the dissected coronary segment.

Also the source of the blood dissecting the coronary wall is controversial. In contrast with the thoracic aorta, there are no vasa vasorum in the coronary arterial wall to potentially account for intramural hematoma. The finding of an intimal tear is quite rare at postmortem in spontaneous coronary dissection, probably because technical difficulties to detect [44] (Fig. 3.32). On the contrary, it is regularly seen in iatrogenic cases complicating catheter maneuvers, like selective coronary angiography, angioplasty, and cannulation of coronary ostia for cardioplegia during surgery. Nonetheless, angiography of coronary dissection typically shows a "binary" appearance (true and false lumen), which clearly suggests an intimal entry into the false lumen. Exceptionally, cystic medial necrosis, similar to that observed in aortic dissection, can be detected (Fig. 3.33). Finally, external factors like trauma or drug abuse should be carefully investigated. In particular, cocaine addiction has been even associated with coronary dissection. The elevated wall stress, due to increased arterial blood pressure from cocaine's inotropic and chronotropic effects combined with its direct vasoconstrictive effect, may be responsible for the formation of an intimal tear and the subsequent dissection of the coronary artery [50].

3.3 Congenital Coronary Artery Anomalies

Anomalies of the origin and course of the major coronary arteries may account of myocardial ischemia and SCD especially during effort [51–56].

In the normal heart, the coronary arteries arise from the left and right anterior sinuses of Valsalva of the aorta, perpendicular to the aortic wall. The pulmonary root, which is anterior and to the left of the aorta, does not interfere with the origin and proximal course of the left and right coronary arteries [57] (Figs. 3.34 and 3.35).

Major anomalies, like the origin of the left or, more rarely, the right coronary artery from the pulmonary trunk (Figs. 3.36 and 3.37), have been reported in cases of juvenile or infant SCD [55]. The origin of a coronary artery from the pulmonary trunk accounts of an aortic–pulmonary fistula: the different resistance between the systemic and pulmonary blood circulation entails a left-to-right shunt with a blood steal from the myocardium, severe myocardial ischemia, and necrosis [58]. The shunt and steal is not present during fetal life, when the systemic and pulmonary resistances are equal. The situation precipitates at birth, at the time of closure of the ductus arteriosus, with the onset of lung respiratory function and fall of pulmonary vascular resistance. Then, the anomalous origin of a coronary artery from the pulmonary trunk may be so severe as to become incompatible with the postnatal blood circulation, because of the ischemic myocardial injury. Cases, however, have been reported with long-term survival as to benefit surgical repair with reconnection of the anomalous coronary artery to the aorta [59, 60].

Other apparently minor, and more frequent, coronary artery anomalies are life-threatening in adolescence and young age. They may be classified into four major categories, with different degrees of certainty (i.e., certain, highly probable, or uncertain) in defining the cause–effect relationship between the anomaly and the SCD event [61]:

1. *Origin of a main coronary artery from the opposite (wrong) sinus.* This is the case of origin of the right coronary artery from the left aortic sinus or origin of the left coronary artery for the right anterior sinus [62–65] (Figs. 3.38 and 3.39). The latter is much more malignant because the anteroseptal and lateral walls of the left ventricle are perfused by this artery, whereas the former has been reported also as incidental finding in noncardiac deaths. They may be well visualized in vivo by coronary angiography or even noninvasively by two-dimensional echocardiography, cardiac magnetic resonance or computed axial tomography [65]. The anomalous origin of the coronary artery from the wrong sinus is a cause of ischemia, especially during effort, through several mechanisms (Figs. 3.40, 3.41, and 3.42):
   (a) An obtuse angle takeoff from the aorta
   (b) A slit-like lumen
   (c) The anomalous vessel running between the aorta and the pulmonary artery
   (d) The intramural aortic course of the proximal anomalous coronary artery

They all contribute to precipitate a discrepancy between coronary blood flow demand during effort and effective coronary blood perfusion across the stenotic proximal coronary segment. Repeated prolonged efforts create focal myocardial ischemic injury that with time precipitates patchy, highly arrhythmogenic fibrotic scars (Fig. 3.43). Combination of acute and chronic myocardial damage is a cocktail of malignant substrate with life-threatening electrical turmoil.

2. *Origin of the left circumflex artery from the right coronary artery or directly from the right sinus of Valsalva* (Fig. 3.44). This is the most frequent coronary anomaly and a source of controversy, because it is usually considered a benign variant. However, cases in which this coronary anatomy pattern was the only abnormality found at autopsy of SCD (Fig. 3.45) have been observed, associated even with myocardial infarction just in the related left lateral myocardial region and in the absence of atherosclerotic obstructive disease [66, 67] (Fig. 3.46).

3. *High takeoff of a coronary artery.* Usually the coronary ostia are located just underneath or above the sino-tubular junction [68] (Fig. 3.35). There are cases of SCD, in which the sole abnormality is an origin of the coronary artery from the tubular part of the aorta, 1–2 cm above the sino-tubular junction [53, 54] (Figs. 3.47 and 3.48). This is usually the case of the right coronary artery, which, by reaching the right AV groove, presents with a vertical course within the aortic tunica media, a condition which clearly impairs coronary blood flow at the time of increased demand during effort, as it is with a coronary artery arising from a wrong sinus.

4. *Myocardial bridge.* Intramyocardial course of a major coronary artery, particularly the left anterior descending branch, is quite common (nearly 30 % of people) as to be considered a variant of normal. There are cases, however, with angina and ECG ST segment alterations, in the absence of other explanation but a "milking effect" at coronary angiography. The intramyocardial course is deep and long, constricted also during diastole, when coronary perfusion occurs [69]. Histologically, the coronary segment is not simply covered by a myocardial fascicle ("bridge") but also surrounded by a sheath of myocardium acting as sphincter [70] (Figs. 3.49 and 3.50).

In the AECVP guidelines for the investigation of SCD, this substrate is classified among those of uncertain significance in terms of risk [61]. Noteworthy, by reviewing with attention the illustrations of reported cases of SCD with myocardial bridge, they were cases of hypertrophic cardiomyopathy with myocardial bridge [71, 72] and now it is well known that myocardial bridge is part of the phenotypic expression of hypertrophic cardiomyopathy [73].

3.4 Image Gallery

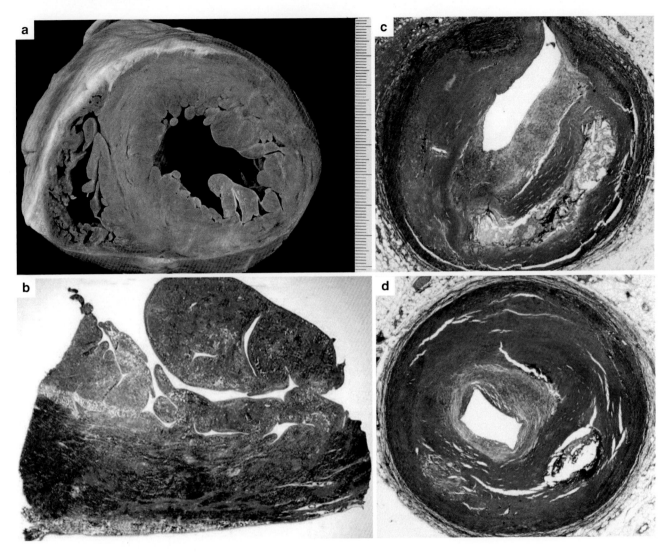

Fig. 3.1 Arrhythmic sudden cardiac death in the adult. A 58-year-old man with previous myocardial infarction due to multivessel atherosclerotic coronary artery disease. (**a**) Transverse section of the heart specimen showing thinning of the posterolateral left ventricular free wall with scarring. (**b**) Subendocardial and patchy transmural replacement-type fibrosis is visible on panoramic histological section of the posterolateral left ventricular free wall (Heidenhain trichrome). (**c**, **d**) Transverse sections of the anterior descending and circumflex branches of the left coronary artery show critical stenosis due to fibro-atheromatous plaques (Heidenhain trichrome)

Fig. 3.2 Arrhythmic sudden
cardiac death in a 30-year-old
man due to atherosclerotic
disease of the proximal left
anterior descending coronary
artery. (**a**) Histology showing
an obstructive eccentric
fibrous plaque at the origin of
the first diagonal branch. Note
the preserved tunica media
(Heidenhain trichrome).
(**b**) Close-up of a, showing a
layer of intimal smooth
muscle cells hyperplasia
(Heidenhain trichrome)

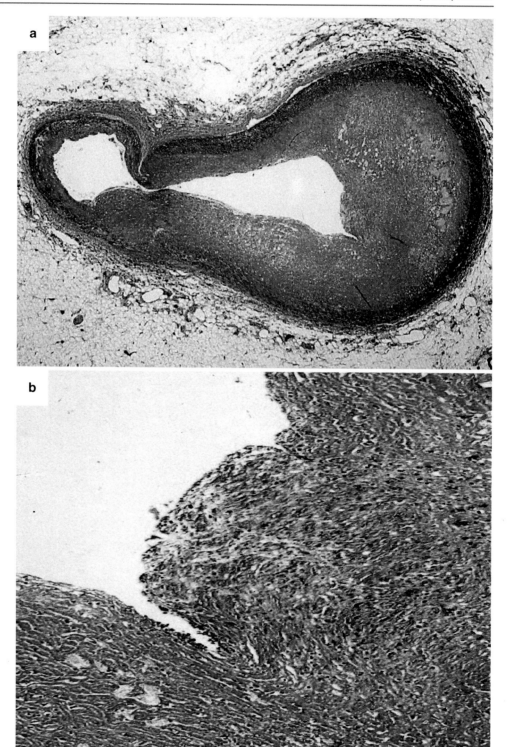

Fig. 3.3 Arrhythmic sudden cardiac death due to vulnerable obstructive atherosclerotic plaque of the proximal left anterior descending coronary artery in the adult. A 56-year-old man. (**a**) Macroscopic examination of the proximal left anterior descending coronary artery showing an eccentric plaque with a *big yellow core* and a *gray fibrous cap*. (**b**) Histology of a vulnerable fibro-atheromatous plaque (Heidenhain trichrome)

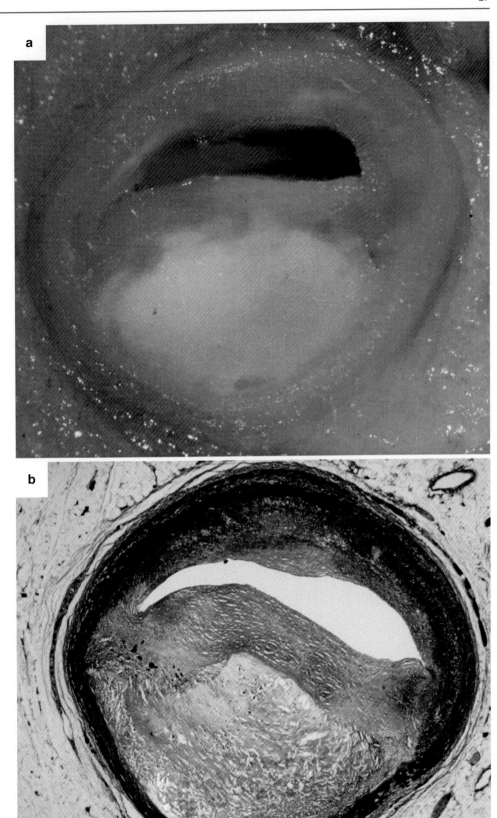

Fig. 3.4 Arrhythmic sudden
cardiac death due to fresh
occlusive thrombosis of the
proximal left anterior
descending coronary artery,
superimposed upon an
eccentric fibro-atheromatous
plaque with a large lipid core
and superficial erosion in a
33-year-old man
(Heidenhain trichrome)

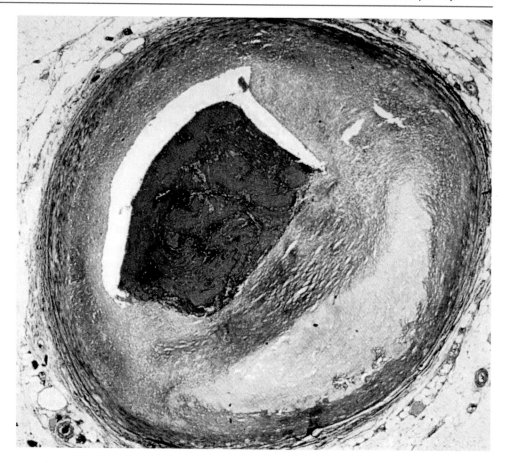

Fig. 3.5 Arrhythmic sudden cardiac death due to single vessel coronary artery disease in a 35-year-old man.
(**a**) An eccentric fibrous fibro-atheromatous plaque, rich in foam cells, is located in the proximal left anterior descending coronary artery (Heidenhain trichrome).
(**b**) Close-up: a layer of intimal smooth muscle cells hyperplasia is visible on the luminal side (Heidenhain trichrome)

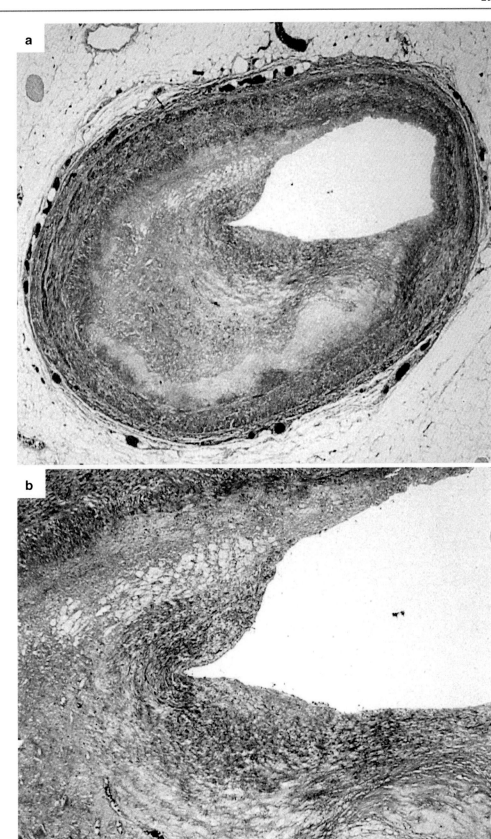

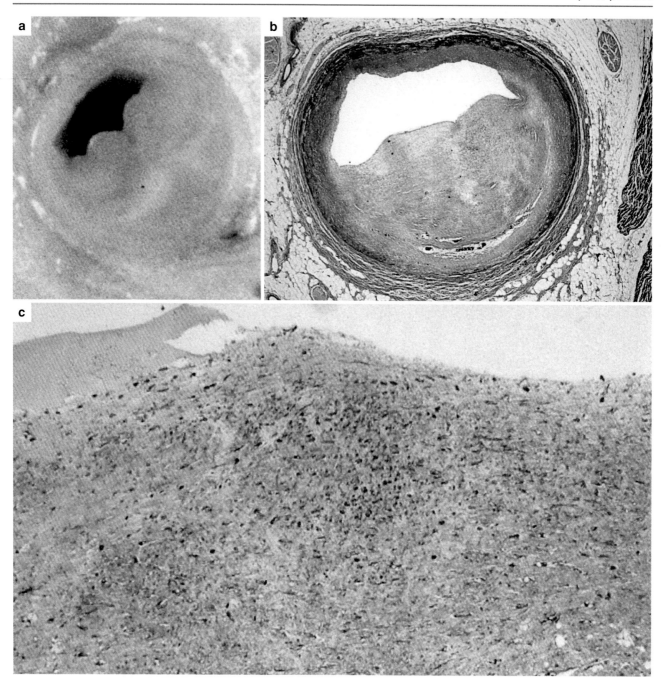

Fig. 3.6 Arrhythmic sudden cardiac death due to single vessel coronary artery disease in a 25-year-old man. (**a**) Macroscopic examination of the proximal left anterior descending coronary artery shows an eccentric, gray plaque. (**b**) At histology, the fibrocellular nature of the plaque, in the absence of a lipid core, is visible (Heidenhain trichrome). (**c**) At higher magnification, note a layer of intimal smooth muscle cells hyperplasia on the luminal side (Heidenhain trichrome)

Fig. 3.7 Immunohistochemistry of an obstructive eccentric fibrocellular plaque located at the level of the proximal left anterior descending coronary artery in a 32-year-old man who died suddenly. (**a**) The intimal cell hyperplasia on the cap of the plaque (*bottom*) consists of smooth muscle cells, since they show an immunoreactivity for smooth muscle actin (SMA) antibody similar to the cells of the media (*top*) (SMA antibody). (**b**) Close-up of the intimal cell hyperplasia, at the top of the plaque (SMA antibody)

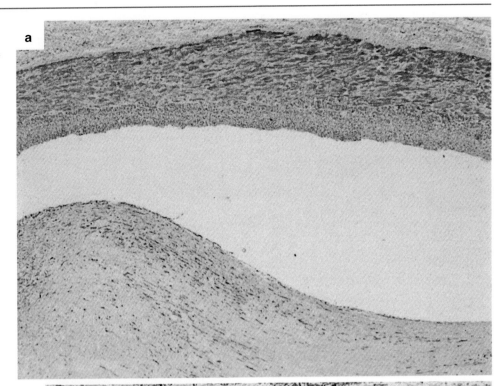

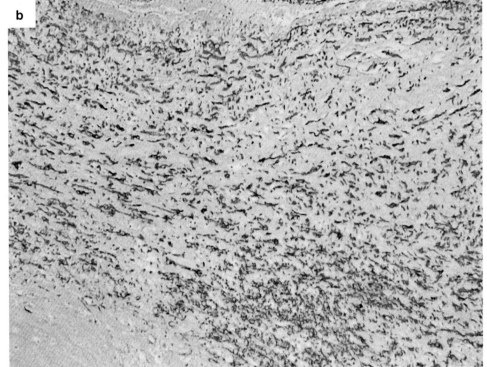

Fig. 3.8 Arrhythmic sudden cardiac death caused by occlusive thrombosis of the left anterior descending coronary artery in a 34-year-old man due to plaque rupture. (**a**) The acute luminal thrombosis is visible upon a fibro-atheromatous plaque (Heidenhain trichrome). (**b**) On the adjacent, parallel, coronary artery section, a rupture at the level of the shoulder region of the thin fibrous cap is visible (Heidenhain trichrome). (**c**) By immunohistochemistry, the fibrous cap appears massively infiltrated by macrophages (CD68 antibody)

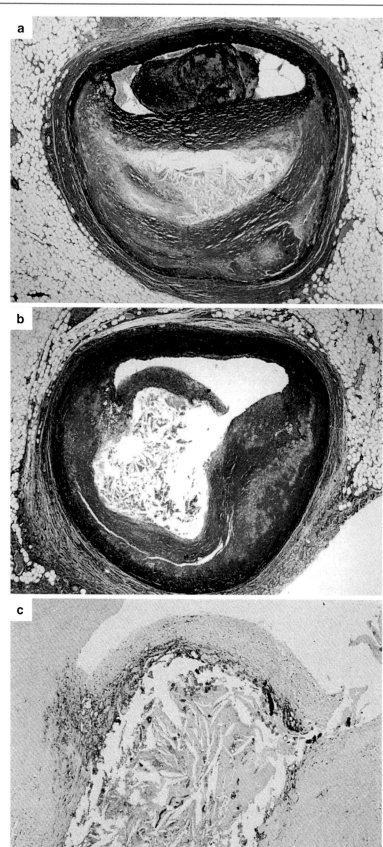

Fig. 3.9 Arrhythmic sudden cardiac death caused by occlusive thrombosis of the left anterior descending coronary artery in the adult, a 55-year-old man with plaque rupture. (**a**) Gross view of the culprit coronary segment showing the acute luminal thrombosis upon a nonobstructive atherosclerotic plaque. (**b**) On the corresponding histological slide of the fibroatheromatous plaque, abundant cholesterol clefts in the necrotic core and the rupture of a thin fibrous cap with occlusive thrombosis are visible (Heidenhain trichrome)

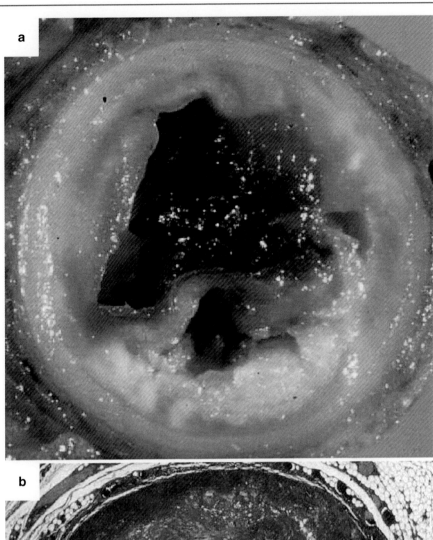

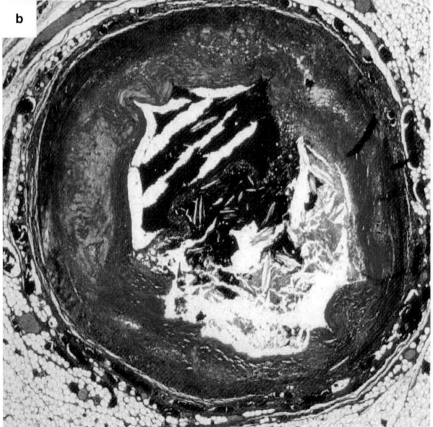

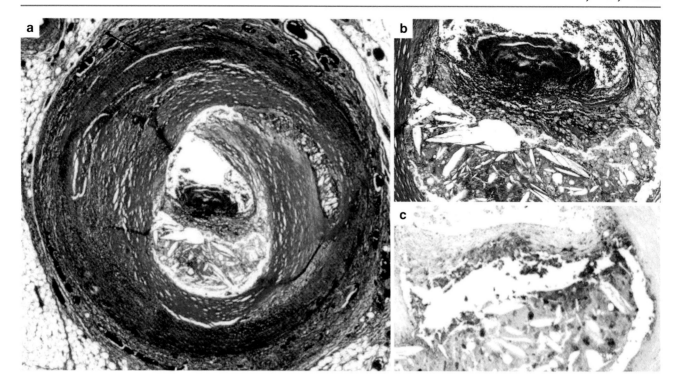

Fig. 3.10 Arrhythmic sudden cardiac death caused by occlusive thrombosis of the left anterior descending coronary artery in the adult, a 60-year-old man with plaque rupture. (**a**) Histological section of the culprit coronary segment showing the acute luminal thrombosis complicating an obstructive fibro-atheromatous plaque with a thin, disrupted, fibrous cap (Heidenhain trichrome). (**b**) Close-up of a, shows abundant cholesterol clefts and hemorrhage in the necrotic core and the thin, disrupted, fibrous cap (Heidenhain trichrome). (**c**) Same field as in (**b**), note the massive infiltration by macrophages of the thin fibrous cap as well as of the necrotic core (CD68 antibody), releasing matrix metalloproteinases

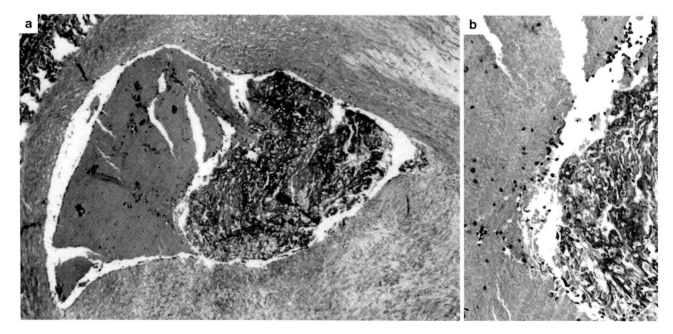

Fig. 3.11 Arrhythmic sudden cardiac death due to occlusive thrombosis of the left anterior descending coronary artery (culprit lesion) in a 40-year-old woman. (**a**) The thrombus is a mixture of platelets (*left*) and fibrin (*right*) entrapping red cells (Heidenhain trichrome). (**b**) Close-up of **a**, showing the border between platelets and fibrin network (Heidenhain trichrome)

Fig. 3.12 Arrhythmic sudden cardiac death due to occlusive thrombosis of the left anterior descending coronary artery with plaque erosion in two 30-year-old men. (**a**, **b**) Fibrocellular, nonobstructive, eccentric atherosclerotic plaques, devoid of lipids, are complicated by occlusive thrombosis, in the absence of fibrous cap rupture (so-called plaque "erosion") (Heidenhain trichrome)

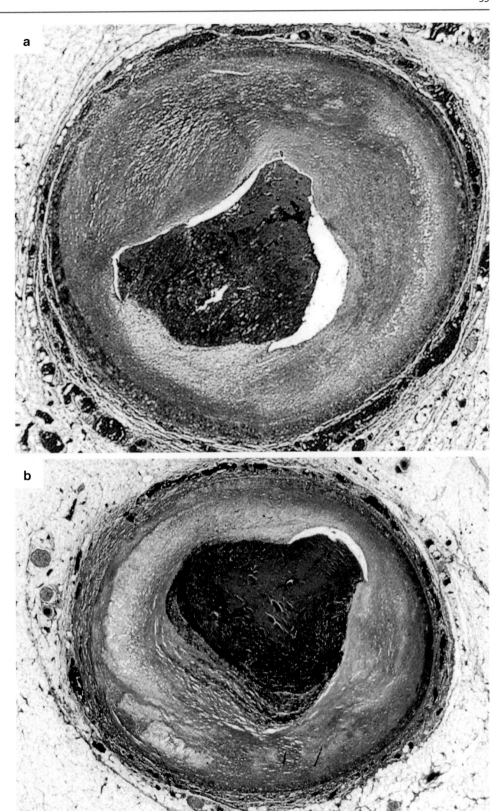

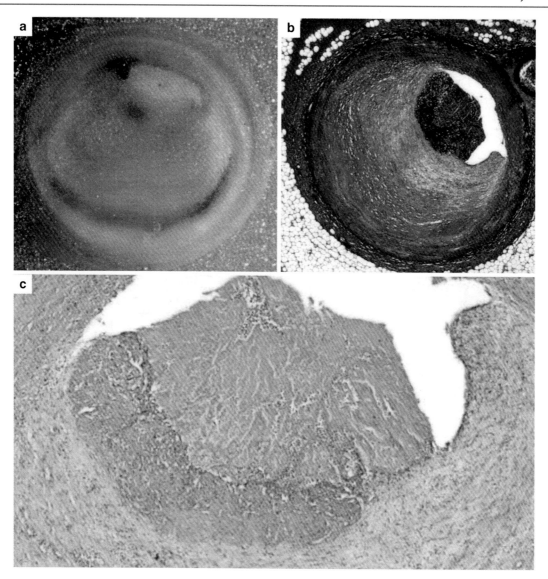

Fig. 3.13 Arrhythmic sudden cardiac death due to occlusive thrombosis of the left anterior descending coronary artery with plaque erosion in a 31-year-old man, with a history of drug abuse (cannabis and cocaine). (**a**) Macroscopic section of the culprit coronary artery showing an occlusive thrombosis upon an eccentric, gray plaque with critical stenosis. (**b**) Corresponding histology with evidence of a fibrocellular atherosclerotic plaque, devoid of lipids, complicated by occlusive thrombosis (Heidenhain trichrome). (**c**) At higher magnification, two separate layers of thrombus deposition are visible, i.e., fresh and subacute with early organization (hematoxylin–eosin)

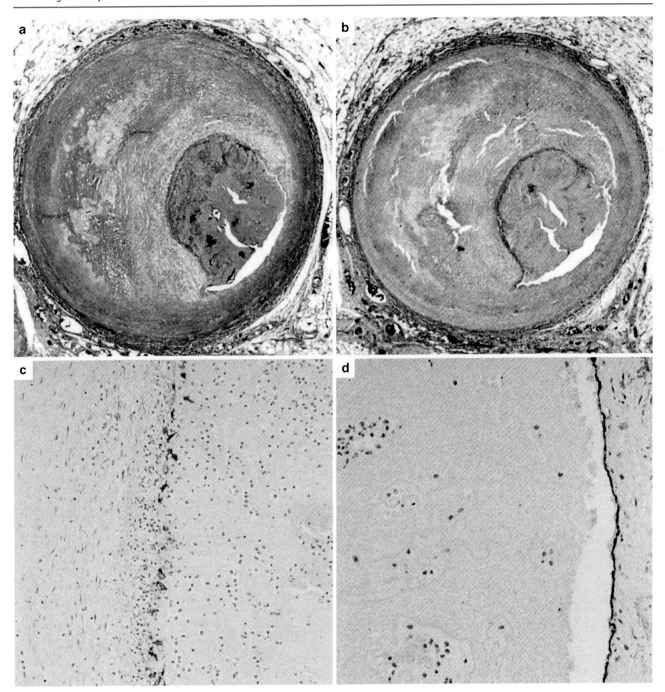

Fig. 3.14 Arrhythmic sudden cardiac death due to occlusive thrombosis of the left anterior descending coronary artery with plaque erosion in a 32-year-old man at rest. (**a**) Histology of the culprit coronary artery shows an eccentric fibrocellular plaque with critical stenosis complicated by occlusive thrombosis (Heidenhain trichrome). (**b**) Same section as **a**, note the inflammatory infiltrate on the intimal surface of the plaque, just underneath the thrombosis (hematoxylin–eosin). (**c**, **d**) At higher magnification, the endothelial layer appears disrupted on the "plaque side" and continuous on the opposite "atherosclerotic free side" of the coronary segment (CD31 antibody)

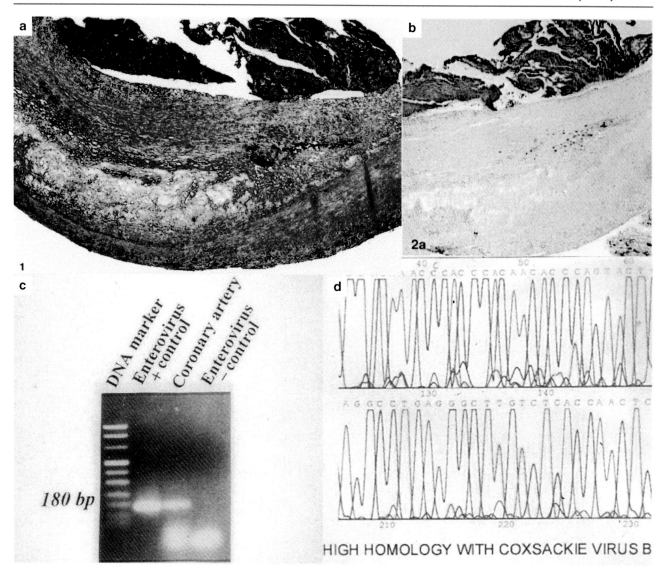

HIGH HOMOLOGY WITH COXSACKIE VIRUS B

Fig. 3.15 Arrhythmic sudden cardiac death due to luminal thrombosis of the left anterior descending coronary artery with plaque erosion in a 26-year-old after an episode of flu. (**a**) Microscopic examination of the culprit coronary artery shows luminal thrombosis upon a fibro-athero-matous non-obstructive eccentric plaque without rupture (Heidenhain trichrome). (**b**) Endothelial erosion in the thrombosed coronary segment (CD31 antibody). (**c**) Agarose gel electrophoresis showing positive result for enterovirus. (**d**) Gene sequencing of enteroviral genome

Fig. 3.16 Arrhythmic sudden cardiac death due to mural thrombosis of the left anterior descending coronary artery with plaque erosion in a 30-year-old man during a soccer game. (**a**) Histological section of the culprit coronary artery showings mural thrombosis complicating an eccentric fibro-atheromatous plaque with a thick, fibrous cap (Heidenhain trichrome). (**b**) Close-up of **a**, note the abundant intimal smooth muscle cells hyperplasia on the luminal side, just underneath the mural thrombus (Heidenhain trichrome)

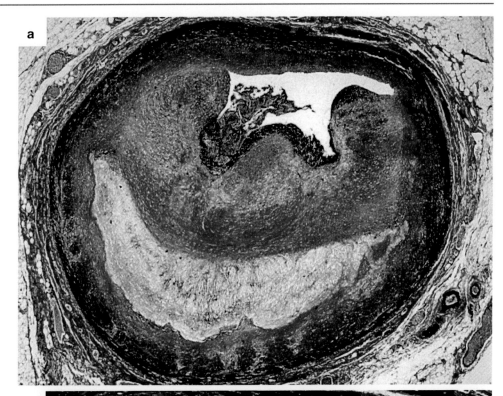

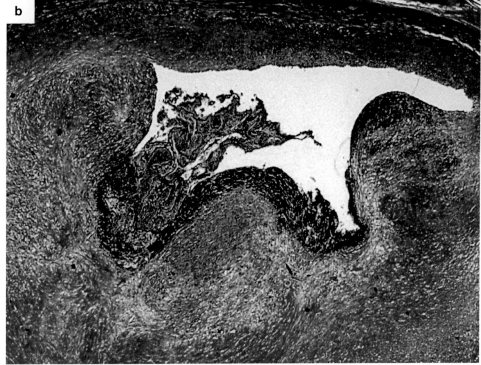

Fig. 3.17 Spontaneous microembolization in the intramural small coronary vessels in the setting of either occlusive or mural thrombosis. (**a**) Diagram showing the detachment of thrombus fragments upon plaque rupture.
(**b**) Thrombotic embolism into a distal intramural small coronary artery (same case as Fig. 3.16, Heidenhain trichrome)

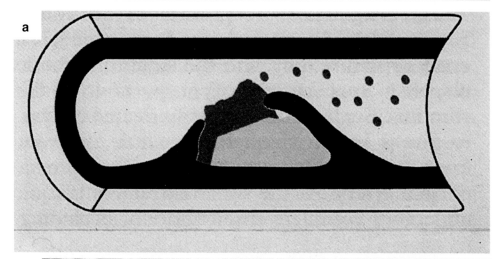

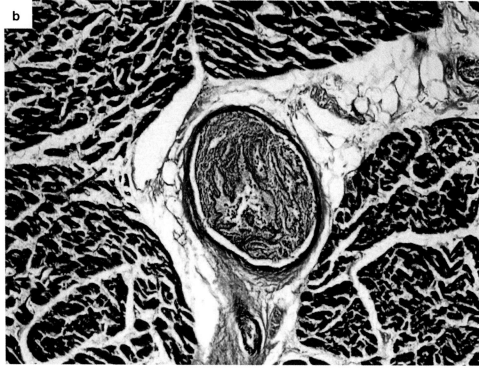

Fig. 3.18 Arrhythmic sudden cardiac death due to "accelerated" atherosclerosis in a 54-year-old man with variant angina. (**a**) Final ECG tracing at Holter monitoring showing ventricular fibrillation preceded by transient ST segment elevation in keeping with ischemia–reperfusion injury. (**b**) Examination of the proximal left anterior descending coronary artery discloses a single obstructive fibrocellular plaque with intimal proliferation of smooth muscle cells enmeshed within mucoid substance. Note the absence of lipid core (Heidenhain trichrome)

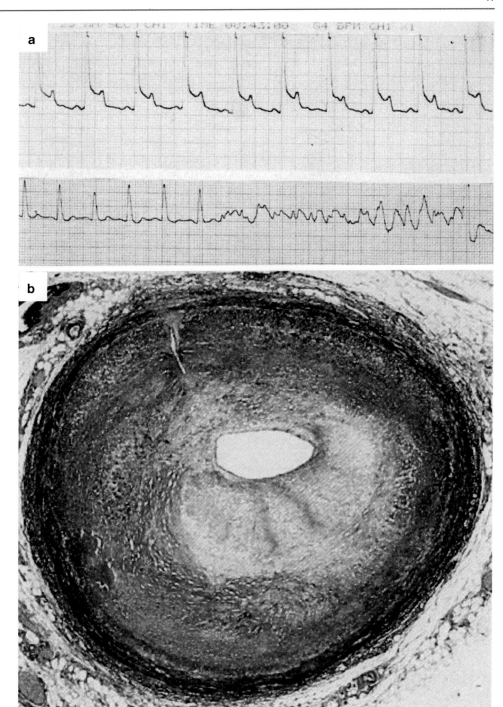

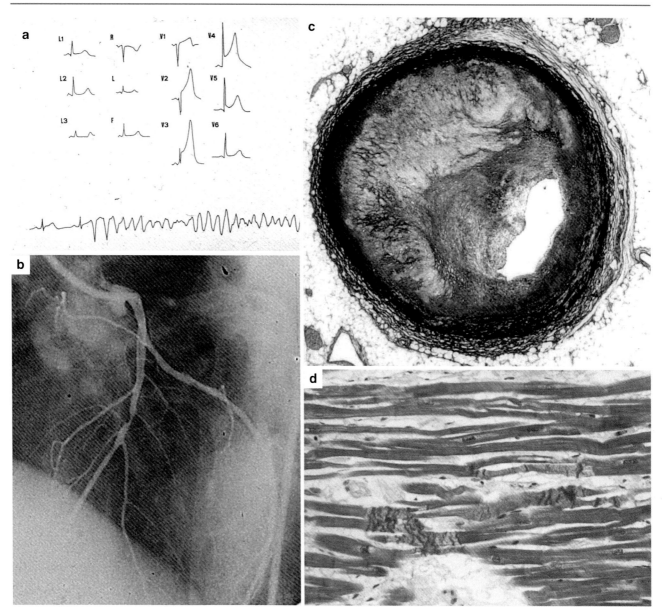

Fig. 3.19 Arrhythmic sudden cardiac death due to "accelerated" atherosclerosis in a 45-year-old man with variant angina. (**a**) Electrocardiographic tracing showing marked ST segment elevation followed by ventricular fibrillation. (**b**) Selective left coronary angiography showing a single obstructive plaque in the mid part of the left anterior descending coronary artery. (**c**) Histology demonstrating a non-

atheromatous, mostly fibrocellular plaque with severe eccentric stenosis and recent intimal smooth muscle cell proliferation; note the preserved tunica media. (**d**) Early signs of ischemic injury with contraction band necrosis in the tributary myocardium are in keeping with transient ischemia and reperfusion (**c** and **d**, Heidenhain trichrome)

Fig. 3.20 Arrhythmic sudden cardiac death due to coronary lumen thrombosis in young cocaine addicts. (**a**) Acute thrombosis of the right coronary artery due to endothelial erosion upon an eccentric fibro-ather-omatous plaque with thick fibrous cap in a 37-year-old man (Heidenhain trichrome). (**b**) Close-up of **a**, showing fibrin deposition on the intimal surface of atherosclerotic plaque (hematoxylin–eosin). (**c**) Same case of (**a** and **b**) showing thromboembolism in the distal branches

(hematoxylin–eosin). (**d**) Acute thrombosis of the left anterior descending branch due to endothelial erosion of an eccentric non-critical fibro-atheromatous plaque in a 28-year-old man (Heidenhain trichrome). (**e**) Acute thrombosis due to fibrous cap rupture of a fibro-atheromatous plaque in the left anterior descending coronary artery in a 45-year-old man (Heidenhain trichrome). (**f**) Recanalized old thrombosis of the right coronary artery (same case of **e**, hematoxylin–eosin)

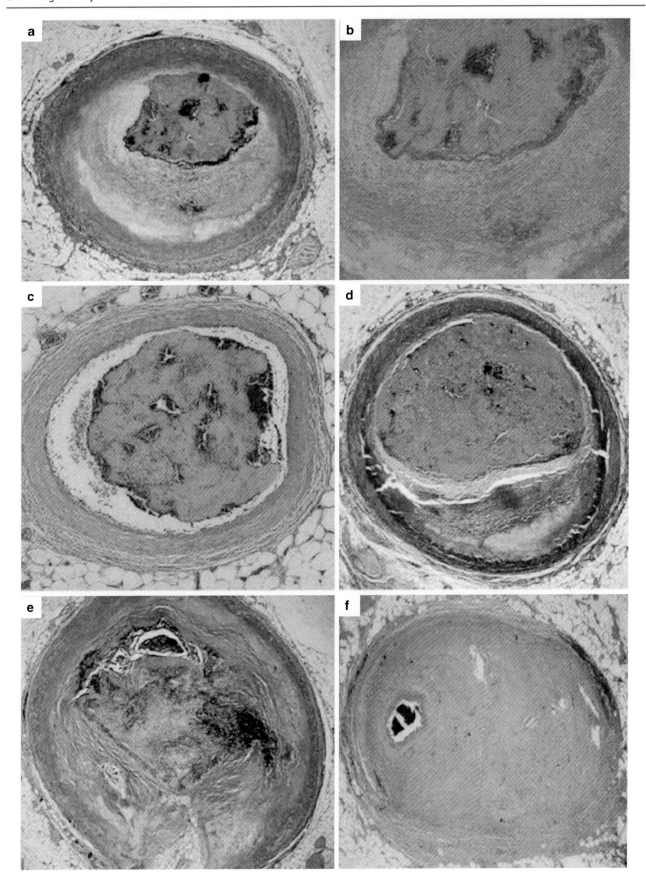

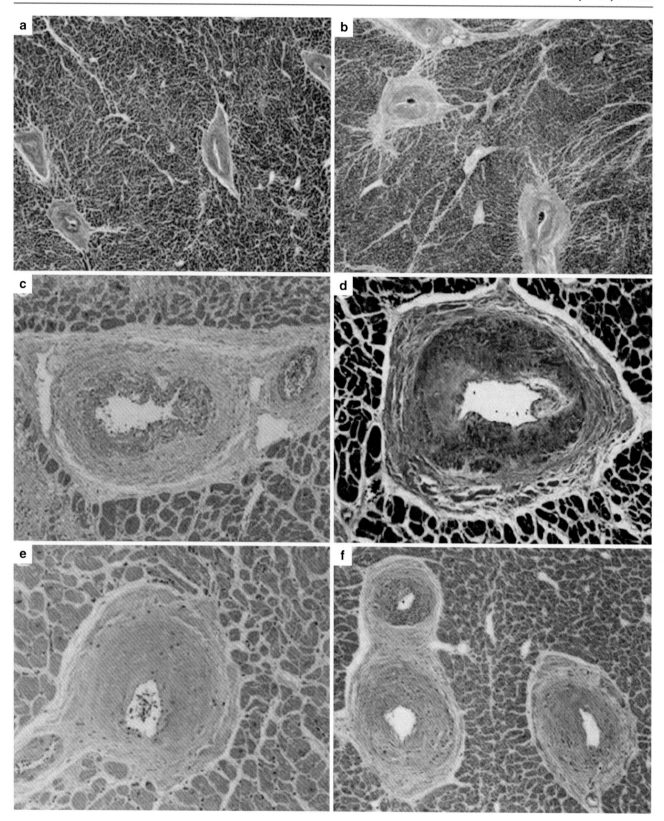

Fig. 3.21 Small vessel disease in cocaine-related sudden cardiac death victims. Note the medial hypertrophy associated with peri-adventitial fibrosis and intimal thickening with narrowed lumen. (**a**) A 21-year-old man (Heidenhain trichrome). (**b**) 28-year-old man (Heidenhain trichrome). (**c**) 28-year-old man (hematoxylin–eosin). (**d**) 34-year-old man (Heidenhain trichrome). (**e**) 37-year-old man (hematoxylin–eosin). (**f**) 45-year-old man (hematoxylin–eosin)

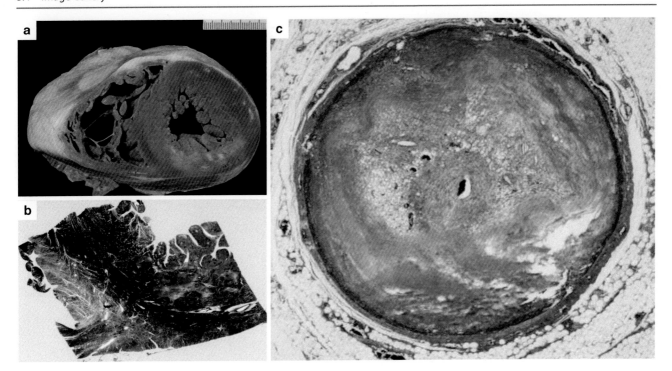

Fig. 3.22 Arrhythmic sudden cardiac death in a 29-year-old soccer player at rest. (**a**) Cross section of the heart showing a subendocardial, posteroseptal healed myocardial infarction. (**b**) Panoramic histology of the posteroseptal area showing replacement-type fibrosis in the subendocardium (Heidenhain trichrome). (**c**) Microscopic examination of the culprit distal left anterior descending coronary artery (recurrent apical) showing healed recanalized luminal thrombotic occlusion (Heidenhain trichrome)

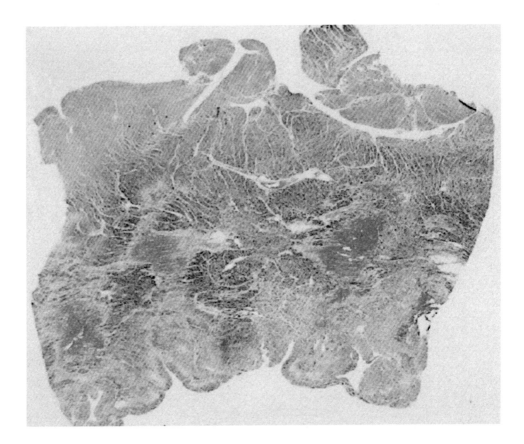

Fig. 3.23 Arrhythmic sudden cardiac death due to previous myocardial infarction in a 43-year-old man. Spots of replacement-type fibrosis are scattered in the anteroseptal wall of the left ventricle, accounting for a zigzag intraventricular impulse propagation (Heidenhain trichrome)

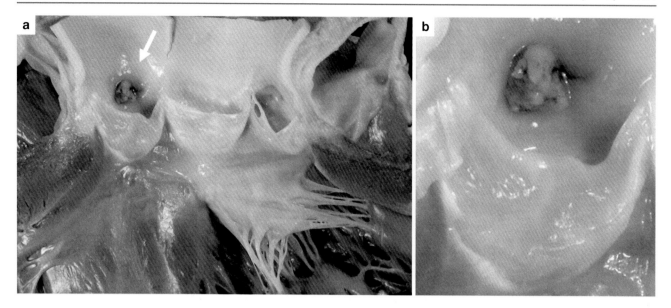

Fig. 3.24 Arrhythmic sudden cardiac death due to coronary thromboembolism in a 25-year-old woman (source of embolism not detected). (**a**) Gross view of the aortic root: note the occlusion of the ostium of the right coronary artery due to a friable thrombotic embolus. (**b**) Close-up of A

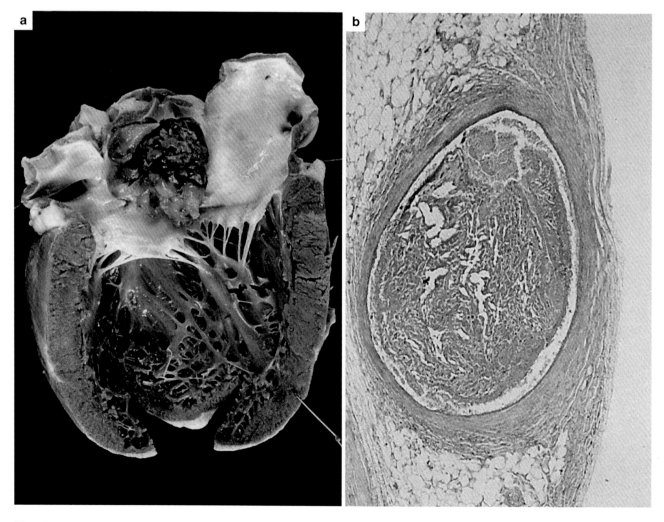

Fig. 3.25 Arrhythmic sudden cardiac death due to coronary neoplastic embolism in a 15-year-old boy with history of malaise and fever. (**a**) Villous myxoma of the left atrial cavity attached on the left side of the atrial septum. (**b**) Histology of the posterior descending coronary artery branch showing neoplastic embolic occlusion by myxoid material (Alcian PAS)

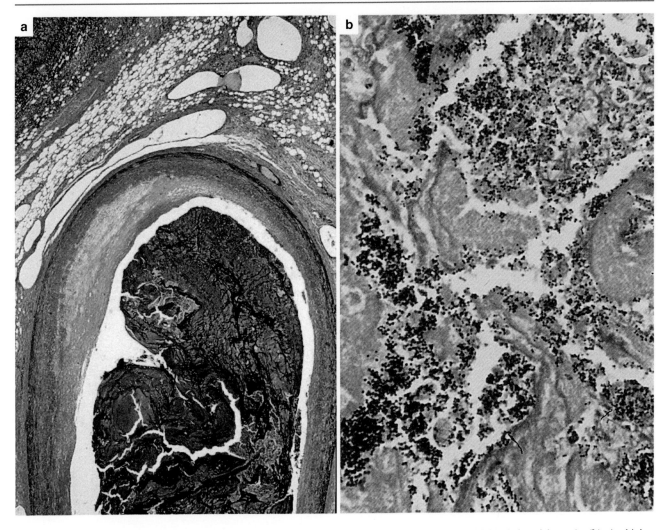

Fig. 3.26 Arrhythmic sudden cardiac death due to coronary septic embolism in a 23-year-old drug addict with aortic valve infective endocarditis. (**a**) Histology of the left main trunk showing the luminal occlusion by a fibrin embolus (Heidenhain trichrome). (**b**) At higher magnification, gram-positive cocci are visible within the fibrin network (Gram)

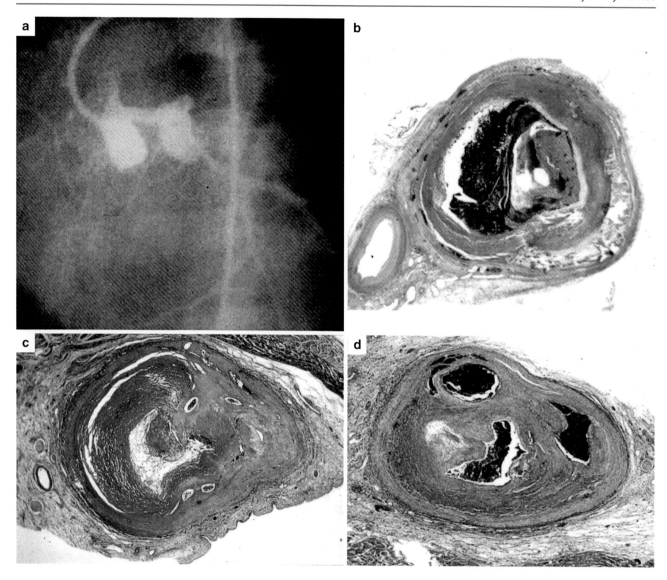

Fig. 3.27 Arrhythmic sudden cardiac death in a 6-year-old boy caused by Kawasaki disease. (**a**) In vivo coronary angiogram: injection in the aortic root reveals huge aneurysm at the bifurcation of the left main trunk. (**b**) Proximal left circumflex artery with aneurysm and thrombosis. (**c**) Right coronary artery with aneurysm. (**d**) Left anterior descending coronary artery with recanalized luminal thrombotic occlusion **b**, **c**, **d** (Heidenhain trichrome)

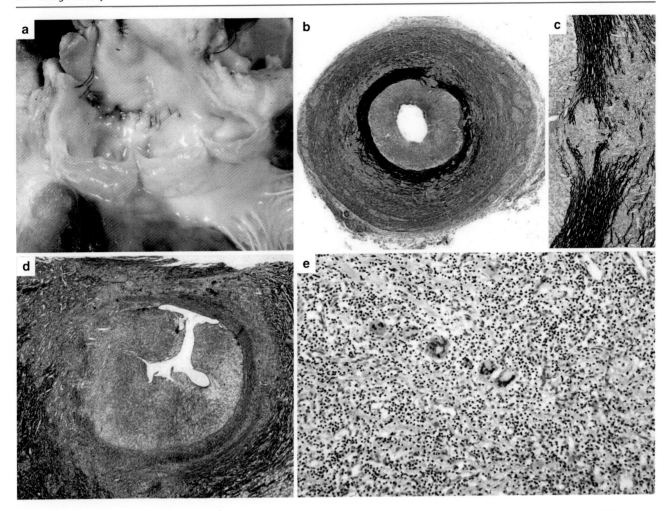

Fig. 3.28 Arrhythmic sudden cardiac death caused by Takayasu disease in a 14-year-old girl. (**a**) Macroscopic examination of the aortic root showing wall thickening and subocclusion of the coronary ostia (note the suture of aortotomy due to emergency bypass surgery after cardiac arrest). (**b**) Histology of the right carotid artery discloses concentric obstructive intimal proliferation, focal disruption of the tunica media, and remarkable adventitial fibrotic thickening (Weigert–van Gieson). (**c**) Close-up of disrupted tunica media (Weigert–van Gieson). (**d**) Histology of the left main coronary trunk showing subocclusion by intimal proliferation with partial disruption of the media (Heidenhain trichrome). (**e**) The inflammatory infiltrate includes giant cells (hematoxylin–eosin)

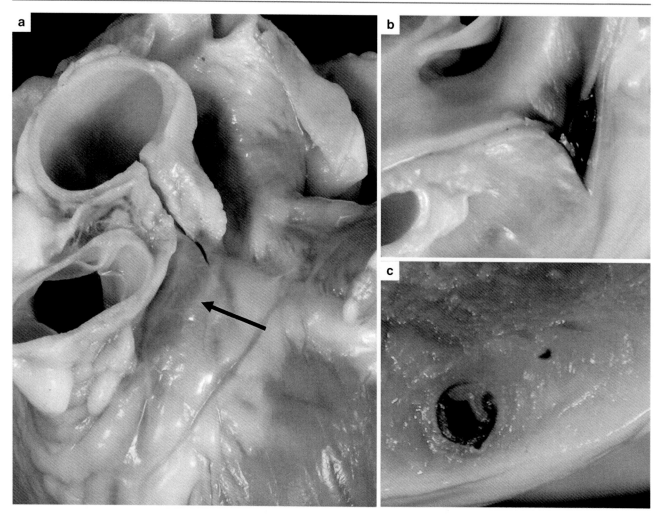

Fig. 3.29 Arrhythmic sudden cardiac death caused by coronary artery dissection in a 34-year-old woman. (**a**) External view of the aortic root: note the bluish color along the course of the left coronary artery (*arrow*: main trunk and left anterior descending branch). (**b**) Opening of the left main trunk from the aorta: note the intramural hematoma. (**c**) Transverse section of the left anterior descending coronary artery shows the virtual true lumen, flattened due to the intramural hematoma in the false lume

Fig. 3.30 Arrhythmic sudden cardiac death caused by coronary artery dissection in a 43-year-old woman. Histology discloses the coronary inner walls flattened by the dissecting hematoma located within the outer tunica media, with true lumen occlusion (**a**, Heidenhain trichrome; **b**, Weigert van Gieson)

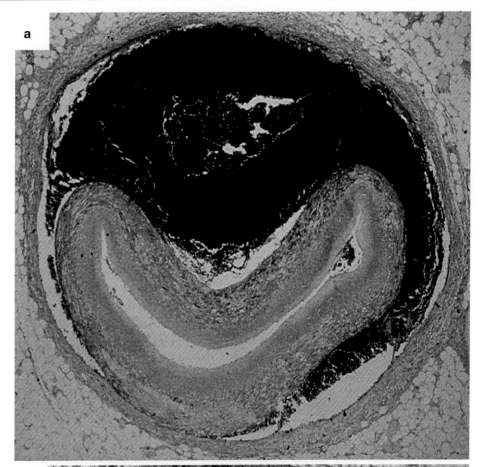

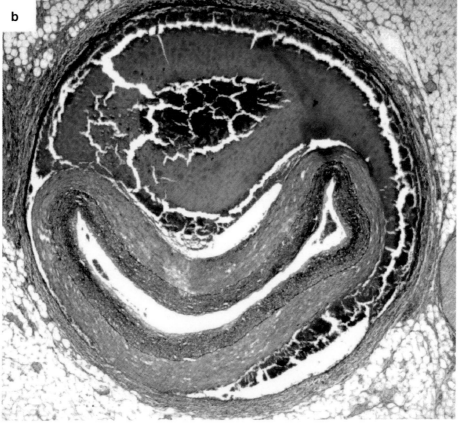

Fig. 3.31 Arrhythmic sudden
cardiac death caused by
coronary artery dissection in a
43-year-old woman.
(**a**) Histology discloses the
coronary inner walls flattened
by the dissecting hematoma
located between the tunica
media and the adventitia, with
true lumen occlusion
(Heidenhain trichrome).
(**b**) Diffuse eosinophilic
infiltrates in the adventitia
(hematoxylin–eosin)

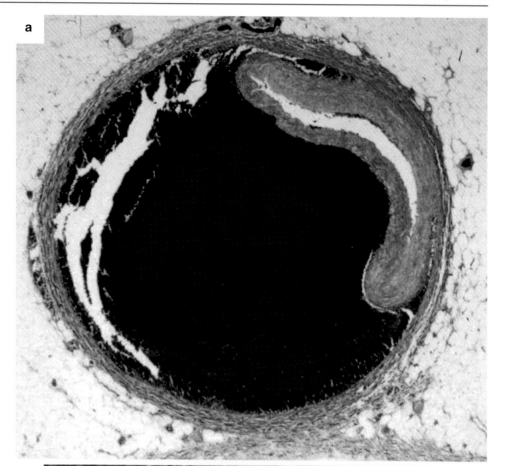

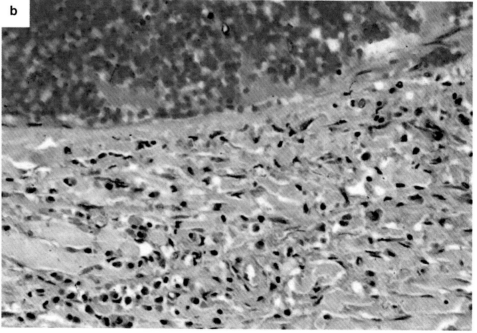

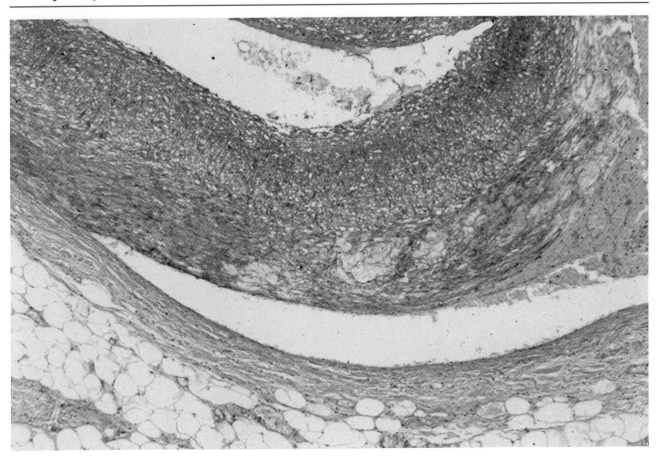

Fig. 3.32 Arrhythmic sudden cardiac death due to spontaneous coronary artery dissection in a 42-year-old woman. Histological section of the dissected left anterior descending coronary artery shows cystic medial necrosis of the tunica media (Alcian PAS)

Fig. 3.33 Acute myocardial
infarction and arrhythmic
sudden cardiac death caused
by coronary artery dissection
in a 48-year-old woman.
(**a**) Serial histological sections
of the dissected left anterior
descending coronary artery
disclose the intimal tear
(Heidenhain trichrome).
(**b**) Close-up of A
(Heidenhain trichrome)

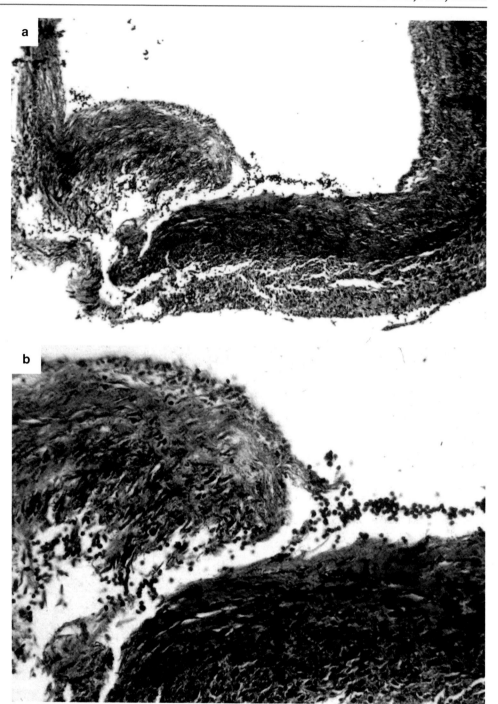

Fig. 3.34 Origin of the coronary arteries in the normal heart, view of the aortic root from above. (**a**) Drawing illustrating the normal origin from the Valsalva sinuses of the aorta facing the pulmonary artery. The pulmonary trunk (PT) does not interfere with the proximal course. (**b**) View of the aortic root of a normal heart specimen from above: note the normal origin of the right (RCA) and left (RCA) coronary arteries, distant from the pulmonary root

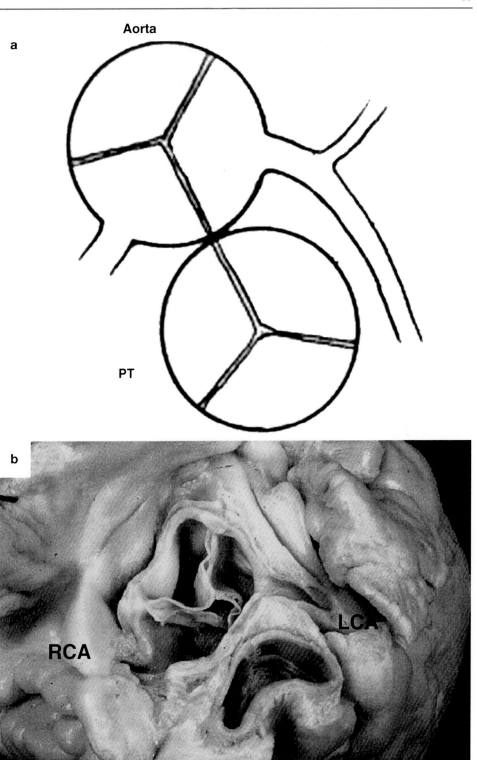

Fig. 3.35 Origin of the coronary arteries in the normal heart, view of the aortic root after opening of the left ventricular outflow tract. (**a**) Diagram illustrating the normal origin from the aorta at the level of the sino-tubular junction: note the normal origin of the right (RCA) and left (LCA) coronary arteries from the corresponding sinuses of Valsalva. (**b**) View of the aortic root of a normal heart

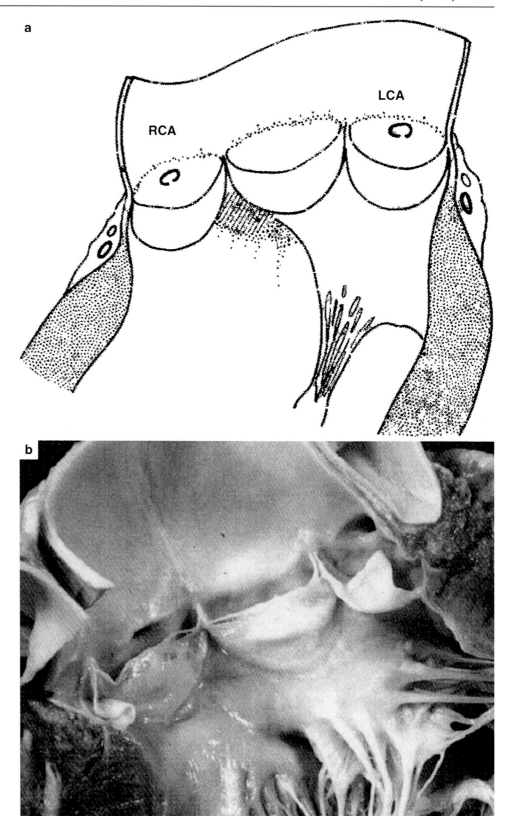

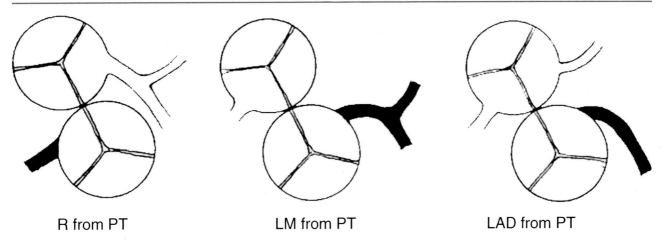

R from PT   LM from PT   LAD from PT

Fig. 3.36 Anomalous origin of the coronary arteries from the pulmonary trunk. Diagrams illustrating right (*R*), left (*LM*) and left anterior descending (*LAD*) origin from the pulmonary trunk (*PT*). These anomalies account for an aorta-to-pulmonary artery fistula, with a left-to-right shunt, and a blood steal from the myocardium ("coronary thieves")

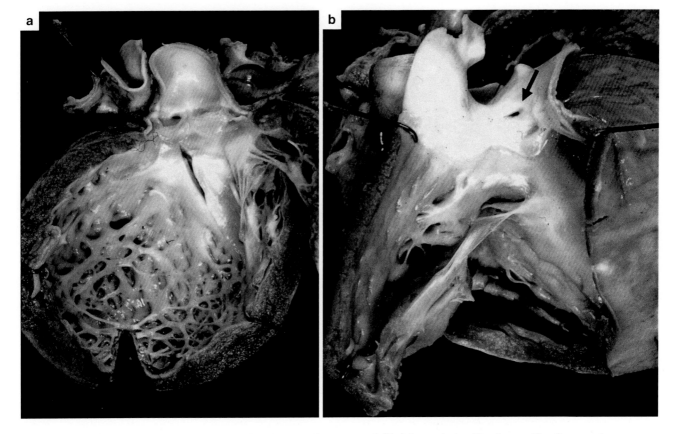

Fig. 3.37 Arrhythmic sudden cardiac death caused by the anomalous origin of the left coronary artery from the pulmonary trunk in a 4-month-old infant. (**a**) View of the left ventricle and aorta; only the right coronary artery ostium is visible at the aortic root. Note the remarkable left ventricular dilatation resulting from previous myocardial infarction with fibroelastic endocardial thickening. (**b**) View of the right ventricle and the pulmonary artery; note the ostium of the left coronary artery located in the pulmonary root (*arrow*)

Fig. 3.38 Anomalous origin
of a coronary artery from the
opposite wrong aortic sinus.
(**a**) Diagram illustrating the
abnormal origin of the left
coronary artery from the right
aortic sinus of Valsalva.
(**b**) Diagram illustrating the
abnormal origin of the right
coronary artery from the left
aortic sinus of Valsalva. In
both instances, the abnormal
proximal coronary segment
runs between the aorta
and pulmonary trunk
(inter-arterial course) with an
acute angle take off

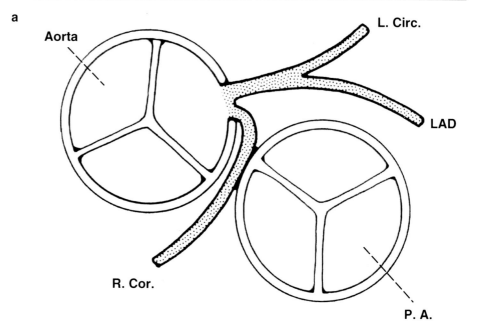

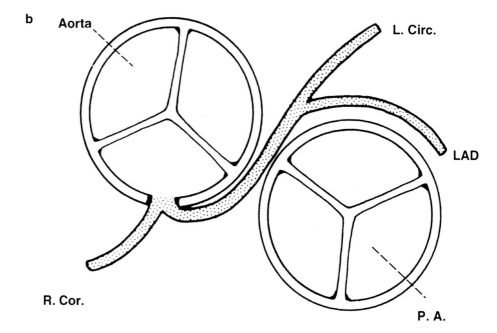

Fig. 3.39 Heart specimens with anomalous origin of a coronary artery from the opposite wrong aortic sinus. (**a**) View of the aortic root showing anomalous origin of the left (*arrow*), with both coronary ostia located in the right aortic sinus (sudden cardiac death during jogging in a 32-year-old woman). (**b**) View of the aortic root showing anomalous origin of the right (*arrow*) with both coronary ostia located in the left aortic sinus (incidental finding at autopsy in a 60-year-old man who died due to hepatitis)

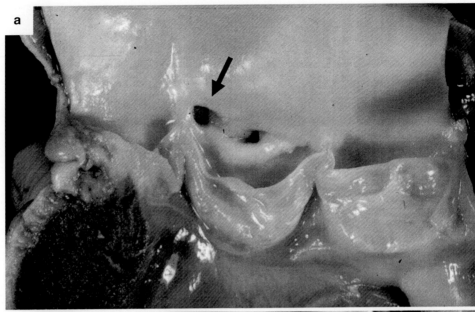

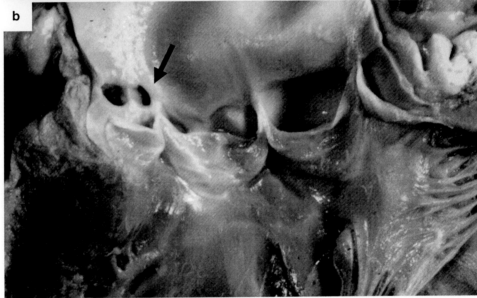

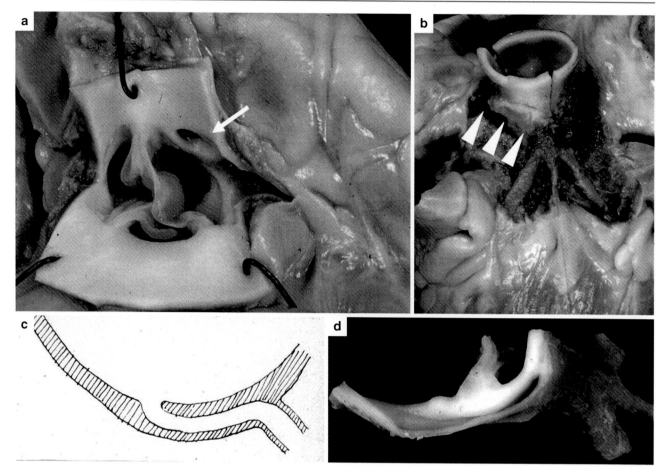

Fig. 3.40 Arrhythmic sudden cardiac death caused by the anomalous origin of the left coronary artery from the right aortic sinus in a 15-year-old soccer player. (**a**) View of the aortic root shows the origin of both the left (*arrow*) and right coronary arteries from the right aortic sinus. (**b**) External view of the aortic root: note the intramural course of the first tract of the anomalous left coronary artery (*arrowheads*), reaching its normal position before dividing into anterior descending, intermediate, and circumflex branches. (**c**, **d**) Diagram and corresponding transverse section of the aortic root at the commissural level: the anomalous left coronary artery shows an intramural aortic course just behind the commissure between the two coronary cusps

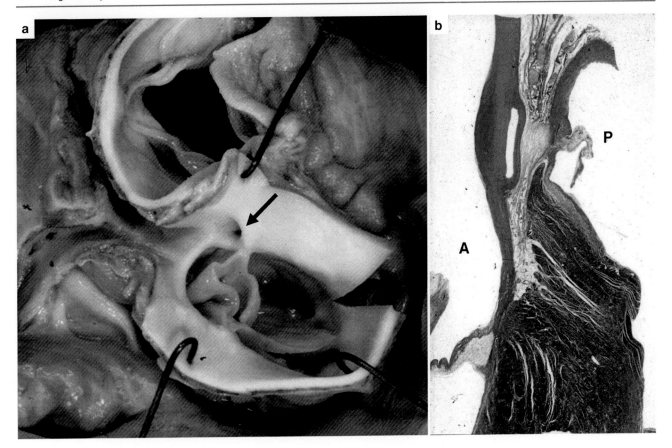

Fig. 3.41 Arrhythmic sudden cardiac death caused by the anomalous origin of the right coronary artery from the left aortic sinus in a 22-year-old soccer player. (**a**) View of the aortic root: note the origin of both the left and right (*arrow*) coronary arteries from the left aortic sinus. (**b**) Histology of the root of the aorta (A) and pulmonary artery (P) reveals the intramural aortic course of the anomalous right coronary artery with slit-like lumen (Heidenhain trichrome)

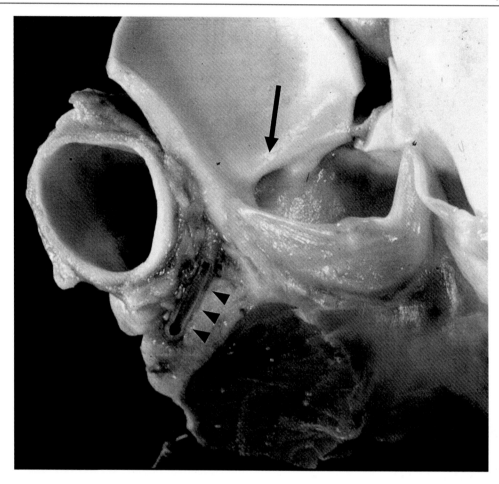

Fig. 3.42 Arrhythmic sudden cardiac death caused by the anomalous origin of the left coronary artery from the right aortic sinus in an 11-year-old soccer player. View of the aortic root shows the origin of both the left (*arrow*) and right coronary arteries from the right aortic sinus. Note the anomalous course (*arrowheads*) of the left coronary artery between the aorta and pulmonary trunk

Fig. 3.43 Histological
section of the left ventricular
myocardium supplied by the
anomalous left coronary
artery (same case as
Fig. 3.40). (**a**) Diffuse
myocyte necrosis and
neutrophilic infiltrates
(hematoxylin–eosin).
(**b**) Multiple patchy areas
of replacement-type fibrosis
within the myocardium
(Heidenhain trichrome)

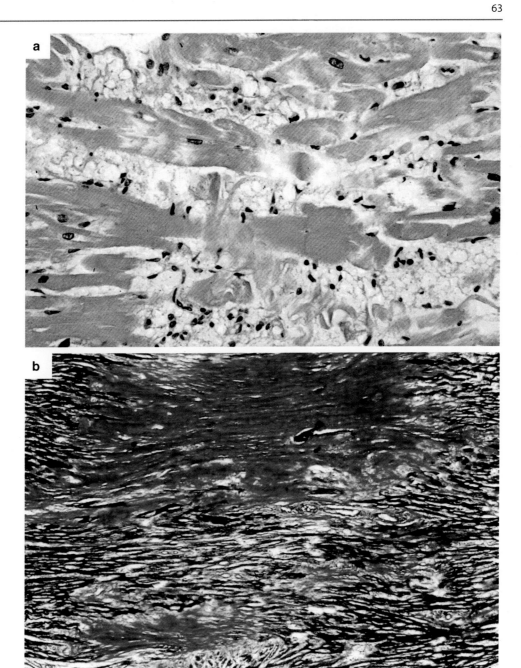

Fig. 3.44 Diagrams illustrating the abnormal origin of the left circumflex (LCx) branch from the right coronary artery (RCA) (or from the right sinus of Valsalva) with isolated origin of the left anterior descending (LAD) branch from the left sinus of Valsalva. (**a**) The anomalous vessel has an acute angle takeoff and a retroaortic course to reach its final destination. (**b**) Dilatation of the aortic root during effort may compress the anomalous coronary artery

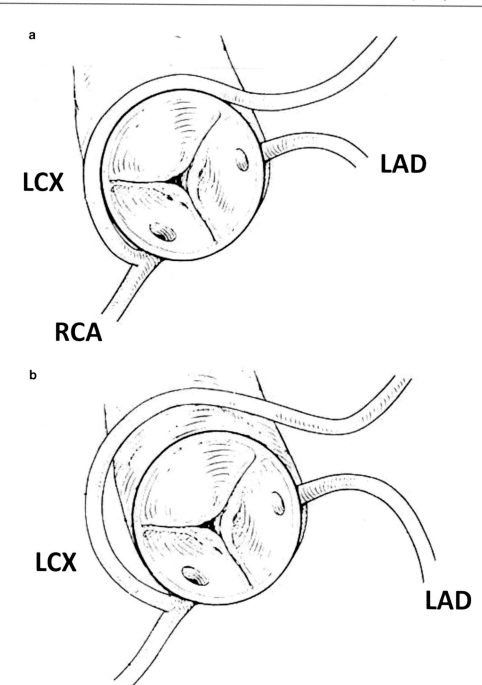

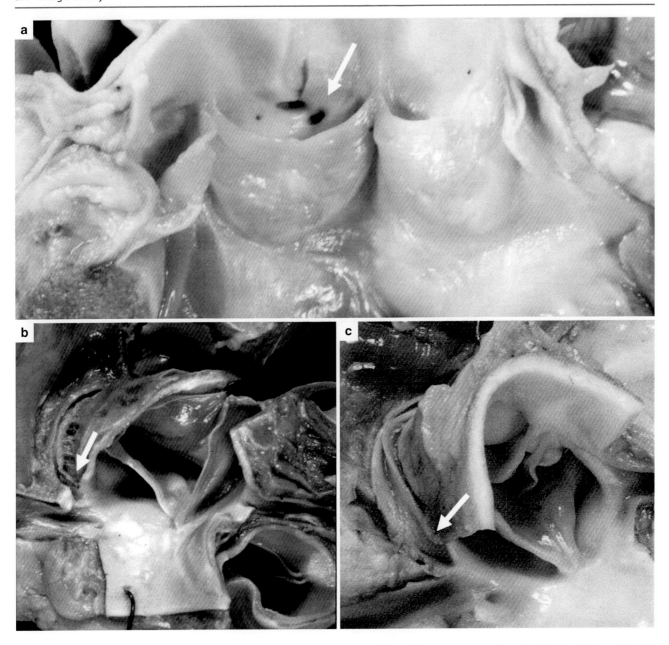

Fig. 3.45 Arrhythmic sudden cardiac death in people with anomalous origin of the left circumflex artery from the right aortic sinus. (**a**) View of the aortic root: note two coronary ostia (*arrow* indicates anomalous left circumflex) in the right sinus of Valsalva, and the normal origin of the left anterior descending coronary artery from the left sinus (19-year-old girl). (**b, c**) Note the retroaortic course of the anomalous left circumflex artery (*arrow*) originating from the right sinus in two additional cases (**b**, 50-year-old man; **c**, 12-year-old boy)

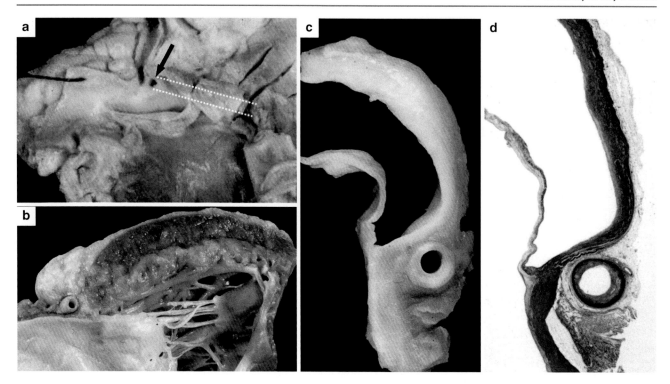

Fig. 3.46 Arrhythmic sudden cardiac death caused by the anomalous origin of the left circumflex artery from the right aortic sinus in a 53-year-old man. (**a**) *Dotted lines* indicate the retroaortic course of the anomalous artery (*arrow* indicates the anomalous origin). (**b**) Gross view of the lateral wall of the patient's left ventricle showing a healed subendocardial myocardial infarction. (**c**) Longitudinal section of the posterior aortic sinus showing the circumflex artery behind. (**d**) Histology of C (Heidenhain trichrome)

Fig. 3.47 High takeoff of the coronary arteries. Diagram illustrating the abnormal origin of a coronary artery (in this diagram the left main trunk – LM) from the tubular portion of the aorta, in contrast with a normal origin (*dotted circle line*) at the sino-tubular junction

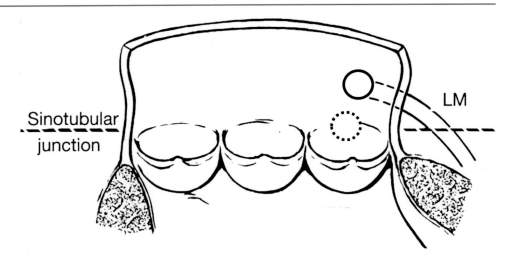

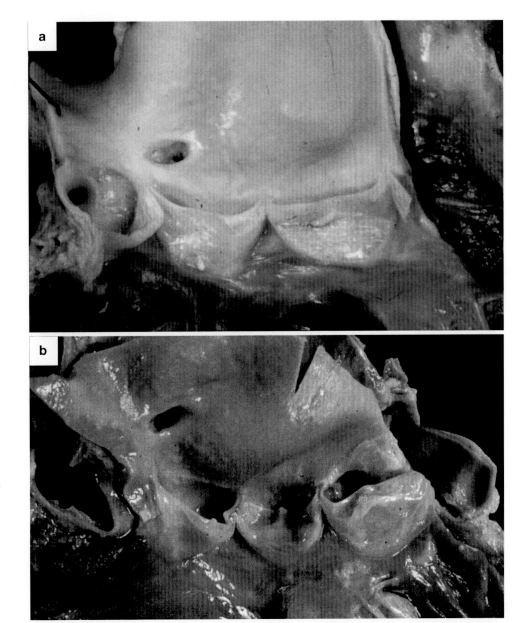

Fig. 3.48 Arrhythmic sudden cardiac death in young people with high takeoff of the right coronary artery as the only structural substrate found at autopsy. Note the funnel-like shape of the first tract with a vertical course to reach the right atrio-ventricular sulcus (**a**, 29-year-old man; **b**, 57-year-old man)

Fig. 3.49 Arrhythmic sudden cardiac death with intramural course of the left anterior descending coronary artery in a 35-year-old athlete during jogging. Note the deep intramural course of the left anterior descending coronary artery with a thick myocardial bridge

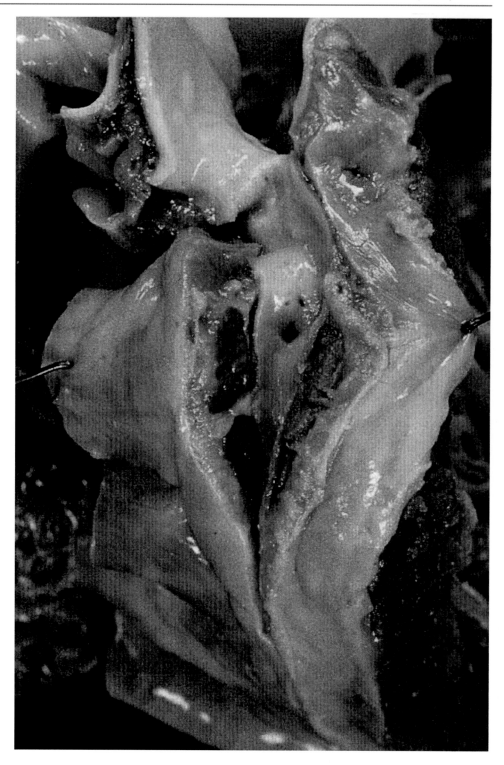

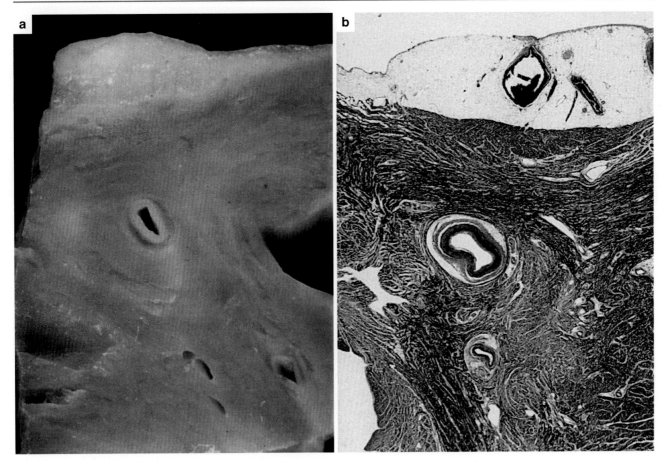

Fig. 3.50 Arrhythmic sudden cardiac death with intramural course of the left anterior descending coronary artery in a 29-year-old man at rest. (**a**) Gross transverse section of the anteroseptal wall showing the deep intramyocardial coronary artery segment. (**b**) At histology, the left intramural anterior descending coronary artery is encircled by a myocardial sheath (Heidenhain trichrome)

References

1. Davies MJ. The investigation of sudden cardiac death. Histopathology. 1999;34:93–8.
2. Thiene G, Carturan E, Corrado D, Basso C. Prevention of sudden cardiac death in the young and in athletes: dream or reality? Cardiovasc Pathol. 2010;19:207–17.
3. Fishbein MC. Cardiac disease and risk of sudden death in the young: the burden of the phenomenon. Cardiovasc Pathol. 2010; 19:326–8.
4. Corrado D, Basso C, Poletti A, Angelini A, Valente M, Thiene G. Sudden death in the young: is coronary thrombosis the major precipitating factor? Circulation. 1994;90:2315–23.
5. Davies MJ, Thomas A. Thrombosis and acute coronary-artery lesions in sudden cardiac ischemic death. N Engl J Med. 1984;310: 1137–40.
6. Davies MJ. Stability and instability: the two faces of coronary atherosclerosis. The Paul Dudley White Lecture, 1995. Circulation. 1996;94:2013–20.
7. Falk E, Nakano M, Bentzon JF, Finn AV, Virmani R. Update on acute coronary syndromes: the pathologists' view. Eur Heart J. 2013;34:719–28.
8. Falk E. Unstable angina with fatal outcome: dynamic coronary thrombosis leading to infarction and/or sudden death: autopsy evidence of recurrent mural thrombosis with peripheral embolization culminating in total vascular occlusion. Circulation. 1985;71:699–708.
9. Henriques de Gouveia R, van der Wal AC, van der Loos CM, Becker AE. Sudden unexpected death in young adults. Discrepancies between initiation of acute plaque complications and the onset of acute coronary death. Eur Heart J. 2002;23:1433–40.
10. Kragel AH, Gertz SD, Roberts WC. Morphologic comparison of frequency and types of acute lesions in the major epicardial coronary arteries in unstable angina pectoris, sudden coronary death and acute myocardial infarction. J Am Coll Cardiol. 1991;18:801–8.
11. Ip JH, Fuster V, Badimon L, Badimon J, Taubman MB, Chesebro JH. Syndromes of accelerated atherosclerosis: role of vascular injury and smooth muscle cell proliferation. J Am Coll Cardiol. 1990;15: 1667–87.
12. Flugelman MY, Virmani R, Correa R, Yu ZX, Farb A, Leon MB, Elami A, Fu YM, Casscells W, Epstein SE. Smooth muscle cell abundance and fibroblast growth factors in coronary lesions of patients with nonfatal unstable angina: a clue to the mechanism of transformation from the stable to the unstable clinical state. Circulation. 1993;88:2493–500.
13. Tavora F, Cresswell N, Li L, Ripple M, Fowler D, Burke A. Sudden coronary death caused by pathologic intimal thickening without atheromatous plaque formation. Cardiovasc Pathol. 2011;20:51–7.
14. Corrado D, Thiene G, Buja GF, Pantaleoni A, Maiolino P. The relationship between growth of atherosclerotic plaques, variant angina and sudden death. Int J Cardiol. 1990;26:361–7.
15. Larsen MK, Nissen PH, Kristensen IB, Jensen HK, Banner J. Sudden cardiac death in young adults: environmental risk factors and genetic aspects of premature atherosclerosis. J Forensic Sci. 2012;57:658–62.
16. van der Wal AC, Becker AE, van der Loos CM, Das PK. Site of intimal rupture or erosion of thrombosed coronary atherosclerotic plaques is characterized by an inflammatory process irrespective of the dominant plaque morphology. Circulation. 1994;89:36–44.
17. Farb A, Burke AP, Tang AL, Liang TY, Mannan P, Smialek J, Virmani R. Coronary plaque erosion without rupture into a lipid core. A frequent cause of coronary thrombosis in sudden coronary death. Circulation. 1996;93:1354–63.
18. Calabrese F, Basso C, Valente M, Thiene G. Coronary thrombosis and sudden death after an enteroviral infection. APMIS. 2003;111: 315–8.
19. Maseri A, Chierchia S. Coronary artery spasm: demonstration, definition, diagnosis and consequences. Prog Cardiovasc Dis. 1982; 25:169–92.
20. Myerburg RJ, Kessler KM, Mallon SM, Cox MM, deMarchena E, Interian Jr A, Castellanos A. Life-threatening ventricular arrhythmia in patients with silent myocardial ischemia due to coronary artery spasm. N Engl J Med. 1992;326:1451–5.
21. Lucena J, Blanco M, Jurado C, Rico A, Salguero M, Vazquez R, Thiene G, Basso C. Cocaine-related sudden death: a prospective investigation in south-west Spain. Eur Heart J. 2010;31:318–29.
22. Montisci M, Thiene G, Ferrara SD, Basso C. Cannabis and cocaine: a lethal cocktail triggering coronary sudden death. Cardiovasc Pathol. 2008;17:344–6.
23. Warnes CA, Roberts WC. Sudden coronary death: relation of amount and distribution of coronary narrowing at necropsy to previous symptoms of myocardial ischemia, left ventricular scarring and heart weight. Am J Cardiol. 1984;54:65–73.
24. Davies MJ. Anatomic features in victims of sudden coronary death. Coronary artery pathology. Circulation. 1992;85(1 Suppl):I19–24.
25. Liberthson RR, Nagel EL, Hirschman JC, Nussenfeld SR. Prehospital ventricular fibrillation: prognosis and follow-up course. N Engl J Med. 1974;29:317–21.
26. Liberthson RR, Nagel EL, Hirshman JC, Nussenfeld SR, Blackbourne BD, Davis JR. Pathophysiologic observations in prehospital ventricular fibrillation and sudden cardiac death. Circulation. 1974;49:790–8.
27. Lovergrove T, Thompson P. The role of acute myocardial infarction in sudden cardiac death: a statistician's nightmare. Am Heart J. 1978;96:711–3.
28. Myerburg RJ, Conde CA, Sung RJ, Mayorga-Cortes A, Mallon SM, Sheps DS, Appel RA, Castellanos A. Clinical, electrophysiologic, and hemodynamic profile of patients resuscitated from prehospital cardiac arrest. Am J Med. 1980;68:568–75.
29. Bezzina CR, Pazoki R, Bardai A, Marsman RF, de Jong JS, Blom MT, Scicluna BP, Jukema JW, Bindraban NR, Lichtner P, Pfeufer A, Bishopric NH, Roden DM, Meitinger T, Chugh SS, Myerburg RJ, Jouven X, Kääb S, Dekker LR, Tan HL, Tanck MW, Wilde AA. Genome-wide association study identifies a susceptibility locus at 21q21 for ventricular fibrillation in acute myocardial infarction. Nat Genet. 2010;42:688–91.
30. Corrado D, Thiene G, Cocco P, Frescura C. Non-atherosclerotic coronary artery disease and sudden death in the young. Br Heart J. 1992;68:601–7.
31. Hill SF, Sheppard MN. Non-atherosclerotic coronary artery disease associated with sudden cardiac death. Heart. 2010;96:1119–25.
32. Thiene G, Basso C. Sudden coronary death–not always atherosclerotic. Heart. 2010;96:1084–5.
33. Basso C, Thiene G, Dalla Volta S. Coronary embolism: a frequently forgotten cause of myocardial infarct and sudden death. G Ital Cardiol. 1992;22:751–60.
34. Basso C, Valente M, Thiene G. Cardiac tumor pathology. New York: Springer Humana Press; 2013 edition.
35. Valente M, Basso C, Thiene G, Bressan M, Stritoni P, Cocco P, Fasoli G. Fibroelastic papilloma: a not-so-benign cardiac tumor. Cardiovasc Pathol. 1992;1:161–6.
36. Basso C, Bottio T, Valente M, Bonato R, Casarotto D, Thiene G. Primary cardiac valve tumours. Heart. 2003;89:1259–60.
37. Bussani R, Silvestri F. Sudden death in a woman with fibroelastoma of the aortic valve chronically occluding the right coronary ostium. Circulation. 1999;100:2204.
38. Byramji A, Gilbert JD, Byard RW. Sudden death as a complication of bacterial endocarditis. Am J Forensic Med Pathol. 2011;32: 140–2.
39. Burns JC, Shike H, Gordon JB, Malhotra A, Schoenwetter M, Kawasaki T. Sequelae of Kawasaki disease in adolescents and young adults. J Am Coll Cardiol. 1996;28:253–7.

40. Daniels LB, Gordon JB, Burns JC. Kawasaki disease: late cardio-vascular sequelae. Curr Opin Cardiol. 2012;27:572–7.

41. Shimizu C, Sood A, Lau HD, Oharaseki T, Takahashi K, Krous HF, Campman S, Burns JC. Cardiovascular pathology in 2 young adults with sudden, unexpected death due to coronary aneurysms from Kawasaki disease in childhood. Cardiovasc Pathol. 2015;24:310–6.

42. Cohle SD, Titus JL, Espinola A, Jachimczyk JA. Sudden unexpected death due to coronary giant cell arteritis. Arch Pathol Lab Med. 1982;106:171–2.

43. Basso C, Baracca E, Zonzin P, Thiene G. Sudden cardiac arrest in a teenager as first manifestation of Takayasu's disease. Int J Cardiol. 1994;43:87–9.

44. Basso C, Morgagni GL, Thiene G. Spontaneous coronary artery dissection: a neglected cause of acute myocardial ischaemia and sudden death. Heart. 1996;75:451–4.

45. Rizzo S, Corrado D, Thiene G, Basso C. Sudden cardiac death in women. G Ital Cardiol. 2012;13:432–9.

46. Tweet MS, Hayes SN, Pitta SR, Simari RD, Lerman A, Lennon RJ, Gersh BJ, Khambatta S, Best PJ, Rihal CS, Gulati R. Clinical features, management, and prognosis of spontaneous coronary artery dissection. Circulation. 2012;126:579–88.

47. Desai S, Sheppard MN. Sudden cardiac death: look closely at the coronaries for spontaneous dissection which can be missed. A study of 9 cases. Am J Forensic Med Pathol. 2012;33:26–9.

48. Robinowitz M, Virmani R, McAllister HA JrU. Spontaneous coronary artery dissection and eosinophilic inflammation: a cause and effect relationship? Am J Med. 1982;72:923–8.

49. Dowling GP, Buja LM. Spontaneous coronary artery dissection occurs with and without periadventitial inflammation. Arch Pathol Lab Med. 1987;111:470–2.

50. Steinhauer JR, Caulfield JB. Spontaneous coronary artery dissection associated with cocaine use: a case report and brief review. Cardiovasc Pathol. 2001;10:141–5.

51. Basso C, Corrado D, Thiene G. Congenital coronary artery anomalies as an important cause of sudden death in the young. Cardiol Rev. 2001;9:312–7.

52. Basso C, Corrado D, Thiene G. Coronary artery anomalies and sudden death. Card Electrophysiol Rev. 2002;6:107–11.

53. Basso C, Frescura C, Corrado D, Muriago M, Angelini A, Daliento L, Thiene G. Congenital heart disease and sudden death in the young. Hum Pathol. 1995;26:1065–72.

54. Frescura C, Basso C, Thiene G, Corrado D, Pennelli T, Angelini A, Daliento L. Anomalous origin of coronary arteries and risk of sudden death: a study based on an autopsy population of congenital heart disease. Hum Pathol. 1998;29:689–95.

55. Roberts WC. Major anomalies of coronary arterial origin seen in adulthood. Am Heart J. 1986;111:941–63.

56. Taylor AJ, Rogan KM, Virmani R. Sudden cardiac death associated with isolated congenital coronary artery anomalies. J Am Coll Cardiol. 1992;20:640–7.

57. Angelini P. Coronary artery anomalies: an entity in search of an identity. Circulation. 2007;115:1296–305.

58. Bland E, White P, Garland J. Congenital anomalies of the coronary arteries. Am Heart J. 1933;8:797–801.

59. Yau JM, Singh R, Halpern EJ, Fischman D. Anomalous origin of the left coronary artery from the pulmonary artery in adults: a comprehensive review of 151 adult cases and a new diagnosis in a 53-year-old woman. Clin Cardiol. 2011;34:204–10.

60. Krexi L, Sheppard MN. Anomalous origin of the left coronary artery from the pulmonary artery (ALCAPA), a forgotten congenital cause of sudden death in the adult. Cardiovasc Pathol. 2013;22:294–7.

61. Basso C, Burke M, Fornes P, Gallagher PJ, de Gouveia RH, Sheppard M, Thiene G, van der Wal A. Guidelines for autopsy investigation of sudden cardiac death. Virchows Arch. 2008;452:11–8.

62. Basso C, Maron BJ, Corrado D, Thiene G. Clinical profile of congenital coronary artery anomalies with origin from the wrong aortic sinus leading to sudden death in young competitive athletes. J Am Coll Cardiol. 2000;35:1493–501.

63. Cheitlin MD, De Castro CM, McAllister HA. Sudden death as a complication of anomalous left coronary origin from the anterior sinus of Valsalva. A not-so-minor congenital anomaly. Circulation. 1974;50:780–7.

64. Liberthson RR, Dinsmore RE, Fallon JT. Aberrant coronary artery origin from the aorta: report of 18 patients, review of the literature and delineation of natural history and management. Circulation. 1979;59:748–54.

65. Lim JC, Beale A, Ramcharitar S. Anomalous origination of a coronary artery from the opposite sinus. Nat Rev Cardiol. 2011;8:706–19.

66. Cohle SD. Circumflex artery from the right coronary sinus: a not-so-benign anomaly. Am J Forensic Med Pathol. 2012;33:107–9.

67. Corrado D, Pennelli T, Piovesana PG, Thiene G. Anomalous origin of the left circumflex coronary artery from the right aortic sinus of Valsalva and sudden death. Cardiovasc Pathol. 1994;3:269–71.

68. Muriago M, Sheppard MN, Ho SY, Anderson RH. Location of the coronary arterial orifices in the normal heart. Clin Anat. 1997;10:297–302.

69. Corban MT, Hung OY, Eshtehardi P, Rasoul-Arzrumly E, McDaniel M, Mekonnen G, Timmins LH, Lutz J, Guyton RA, Samady H. Myocardial bridging: contemporary understanding of pathophysiology with implications for diagnostic and therapeutic strategies. J Am Coll Cardiol. 2014;63:2346–55.

70. Ferreira AG, Trotter SE, Konig B, Ferreira AG, Trotter SE, Konig B. Myocardial bridges: morphological and functional aspects. Br Heart J. 1991;66:364–7.

71. Morales AR, Romanelli R, Boucek RJ. The mural left anterior descending coronary artery, strenuous exercise and sudden death. Circulation. 1980;62:230–7.

72. Gori F, Basso C, Thiene G. Myocardial infarction in a patient with hypertrophic cardiomyopathy. N Engl J Med. 2000;342:593–4.

73. Basso C, Thiene G, Mackey-Bojack S, Frigo AC, Corrado D, Maron BJ. Myocardial bridging, a frequent component of the hypertrophic cardiomyopathy phenotype, lacks systematic association with sudden cardiac death. Eur Heart J. 2009;30:1627–34.

Cardiomyopathies

4

An abrupt electrical turmoil precipitating ventricular fibrillation and cardiac arrest is a frequent complication of cardiomyopathies, whether overt or concealed, because they have an arrhythmogenic myocardial substrate.

When dealing with cardiomyopathies at risk of SCD, according to the World Health Organization, American Heart Association, and European Society of Cardiology definition of cardiomyopathies [1–3], we refer mostly to hypertrophic (HCM) and arrhythmogenic (AC) cardiomyopathies, which are often compatible with normal mechanical function, which is essential for sport activity, but are quite vulnerable in terms of electrical stability. Dilated and restrictive cardiomyopathies unlikely cope with effort performance, because of dyspnea and fatigue, and are an exceptional cause of unexpected SCD in the young and athletes.

4.1 Hypertrophic Cardiomyopathy

It is a major cause of SCD during effort and thus the leading cause of cardiac arrest in athletes in countries such as the United States, where ECG is not employed at the preparticipation screening [4–6]. It is a genetically determined disease, with autosomal dominant pattern of inheritance, mostly due to mutations of genes encoding sarcomeric proteins, and characterized by asymmetrical hypertrophy of the left ventricle, usually septal or apical [7, 8] (Figs. 4.1 and 4.2). Concentric, symmetrical hypertrophy may be also observed.

In case of asymmetrical septal hypertrophy, a fibrous endocardial plaque is usually present in the subaortic position, as a consequence of the friction of the anterior mitral leaflet with the endocardium of the ventricular septum, due to systolic anterior motion of the leaflet, which itself appears thickened (Figs. 4.2 and 4.3).

The histology discloses myocardial disarray, with variously oriented cardiomyocytes crossing each other (either single cell or fascicular), cardiomyocyte hypertrophy with bizarre nuclei, interstitial fibrosis, and dysplastic and frequently obstructed, intramural small arteries [9–16] (Fig. 4.4).

There are several structural substrates which explain why HCM is highly arrhythmogenic and at risk of life-threatening ventricular arrhythmias and SCD:

1. Hypertrophy, which may be so huge as the heart can weigh up to 1000 g. Wall thickness greater than 30 mm is considered one of the major risk factors of SCD.
2. Myocardial disarray, with twirling of cardiomyocytes, an ideal substrate for reentry of the electric impulse transmission and onset of ventricular arrhythmias [14, 15].
3. Fibrous scars, ischemic in origin, mostly due to impaired coronary flow reserve because of cardiac hypertrophy and myocardial restrictivity, with compression of small intramural coronary arteries during the diastole [15] (Figs. 4.5, 4.6, and 4.7); organic small vessel obstructive disease may also contribute (Fig. 4.4).
4. Myocardial bridge of the left anterior descending coronary artery, a peculiar component of the phenotype of HCM, much more frequent than in the normal heart. However, a significant relation between myocardial bridge and SCD has not been definitely proven in HCM [15, 16] (Figs. 4.7, 4.8, and 4.9).

Observation of scars within the hypertrophy is almost regular at autopsy of cases with HCM and SCD, even when the wall thickness and the heart weight are not particularly increased [16]. In support of the ischemic etiology of replacement-type fibrosis, all the stages of ischemic myocardial injury are seen in the hearts of people dying suddenly with HCM, including interstitial edema, myocyte coagulative necrosis, neutrophilic infiltrates, and myocytolysis, eventually leading to scarring [15] (Fig. 4.10). By the way, the progressive scarring accounts for the evolution of HCM into a dilated, end-stage form [17].

Disarray and replacement-type fibrosis appear to be a malignant arrhythmic combination. Replacement-type

© Springer-Verlag Milan 2016
G. Thiene et al., *Sudden Cardiac Death in the Young and Athletes: Text Atlas of Pathology and Clinical Correlates*,
DOI 10.1007/978-88-470-5776-0_4

fibrosis is easily identified in vivo by contrast-enhanced cardiac magnetic resonance imaging [18].

A so-called idiopathic left ventricular hypertrophy has been reported in young people and athletes who died suddenly [4–6]. The degree of hypertrophy is beyond that seen in the cardiac hypertrophy of the trained athlete, with left ventricular thickness exceeding 15 or 16 mm. It is a diagnosis by exclusion, after ruling out other conditions that would predispose to left ventricular hypertrophy (e.g., aortic valve stenosis, isthmic aortic coarctation, systemic hypertension). Unlike HCM, idiopathic left ventricular hypertrophy is concentric and symmetric and there is no evidence of subaortic plaque and mitral valve disease, myocardial disarray, and familial transmission. Whether this condition should be considered a distinct entity at risk of SCD is still a matter of debate, and differential diagnosis with "athlete heart" remains a challenge not only in the clinical setting but also at postmortem [19–21].

4.2 Arrhythmogenic Cardiomyopathy

It is the leading nonischemic cause of SCD in the young and in the athletes in Italy [22, 23]. In contrast with HCM, which is a sarcomeric disease mostly affecting the left ventricle, AC is a desmosomal disease and has been viewed as a disease of the right ventricle [22–30]. The fibrofatty replacement starts from the subepicardium and deepens as a wave-front phenomenon, reaching the subendocardium, to become transmural [22, 31, 32]. In SCD series, both segmental (Figs. 4.11 and 4.12) and diffuse (Figs. 4.13 and 4.14) forms of AC are described and even cases with early stages of myocardial injury (Fig. 4.15), preceding the mature fibrofatty tissue [22, 24, 31–35]. Biventricular or even isolated or dominant left ventricular forms have also been reported [31, 32, 35–37] (Figs. 4.16 and 4.17). Left ventricular free wall involvement has been observed in up to 70 % of autopsy reports [31, 32], whereas the ventricular septum only in 20 % [31]. In the left ventricle, the subepicardium of the posterolateral wall is typically affected. When the biventricular involvement is diffuse, AC may mimic dilated cardiomyopathy with congestive heart failure, so severe as to require cardiac transplantation. Cases with predominant fatty tissue replacement with preserved wall thickness or even pseudo-hypertrophy do also exist (Fig. 4.18). However, isolated fatty tissue at postmortem cannot be regarded as a pathognomonic feature of the disease [19, 38], in order to avoid a misdiagnosis of AC at autopsy, with forensic and preventive implications, since the postmortem diagnosis must guide cascade investigation of family members [39].

Endomyocardial biopsy is frequently employed to detect fibrofatty replacement in vivo and an amount of residual myocardium less than 60 % is considered diagnostic [40]. Clinical diagnosis is challenging and there is no single gold standard [41]. Typically, the ECG discloses depolarization abnormalities, QRS widening, epsilon waves, and repolarization changes with inverted T waves on precordial leads. In the classical variant, ventricular arrhythmias present a left bundle branch block morphology indicating the right ventricular origin. Low voltage areas by electro-anatomic mapping and late enhancement by contrast cardiac magnetic resonance are now very helpful clinical imaging surrogates of myocardial atrophy [42, 43].

The pathobiological phenomenon consists of a transmural fibrofatty replacement of the ventricular free wall, as a repair consequence of a progressive cardiomyocyte death, either by necrosis or apoptosis [44, 45] (Fig. 4.19). In advanced forms, the myocardium may almost disappear and the free wall looks parchment like. This process accounts for the dilatation of the ventricular cavity and the development of wall aneurysms. In contrast with HCM, where the cardiomyocyte death is mostly ischemic in origin because of impairment of microcirculation due to hypertrophy and wall stiffness constricting the small arteries, in AC, cell death with myocardial loss is genetically determined, due to cell junction vulnerability [44]. AC is indeed a genetic disorder of desmosomes [24–30, 46, 47]. Mutations of genes encoding desmosomal proteins account for a vulnerable intercalated disk, which appears disrupted at electron microscopy [48, 49]. Stretch, due to increased ventricular preload during effort, facilitates both cell death and onset of arrhythmias. Although AC is genetically determined, there is an age and gender related penetrance of the phenotype and SCD typically occurs during adolescence or early adulthood, even as first manifestation of the disease [24–26, 50, 51].

The following substrates of the disease should be considered arrhythmogenic [51]:

1. Fibrofatty replacement of the myocardium, which explains the QRS widening and postexcitation epsilon wave as well as inverted T waves in precordial leads at the ECG. Like in ischemic scars, fibrofatty replacement hinders and delays the intraventricular electrical impulse transmission, thus facilitating reentry phenomena.
2. Development of aneurysms in the right ventricular free wall, which further favors reentry mechanisms for onset of ventricular arrhythmias of left bundle branch block morphology.
3. Dilatation of the right ventricular cavity, especially with chamber overload during effort, with further slowdown of the intraventricular conduction.

4. Inflammatory noninfectious infiltrates ("myocarditis"), most probably as a reaction to spontaneous cardiomyocyte death (Fig. 4.19). They have been reported at histology in up to 75 % of autopsy cases [31, 44, 52]. Bursts of cardiomyocyte necrosis with reactive inflammation may trigger life-threatening arrhythmias. This is most probably the explanation why they are so frequently observed at postmortem in subjects who had died suddenly.

It is still a matter of debate whether electrical instability at risk of SCD might occur also in the pre-phenotypic stage of the disease, before structural abnormalities of the myocardium, due to a cross-talk between mechanical junction and ion channels. Experimental studies demonstrated that intercellular space widening at the level of the intercalated disk and a concomitant reduction in action potential upstroke velocity, as a consequence of lower sodium current density, lead to slowed conduction and increased arrhythmia susceptibility at disease stages preceding the onset of necrosis and replacement fibrosis [49]. However, no single SCD case has been reported so far in the pre-phenotypic stage of AC.

4.3   Image Gallery

Fig. 4.1 Arrhythmic sudden cardiac death due to hypertrophic cardiomyopathy in a 37-year-old man during exercise. (**a**) Parasternal long-axis section of the heart shows asymmetric septal hypertrophy as compared to the posterior left ventricular wall. Note the absence of endocardial fibrous plaque. (**b**) At histology, extensive myocardial disarray and interstitial fibrosis (Heidenhain trichrome)

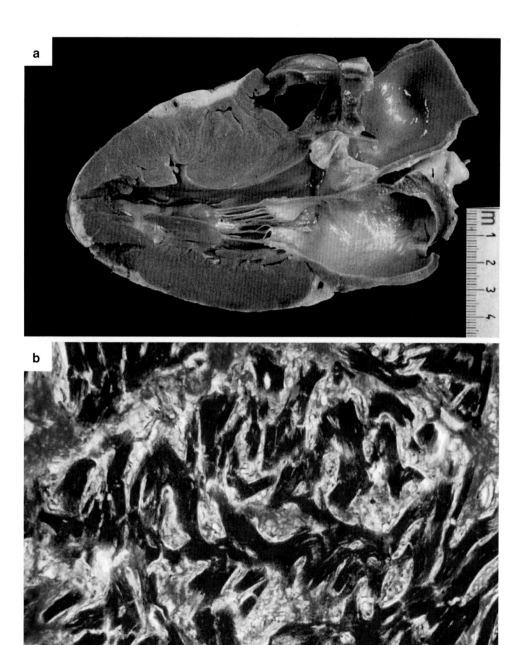

Fig. 4.2 Arrhythmic sudden cardiac death on effort due to hypertrophic cardiomyopathy in a 17-year-old athlete. (**a**) Parasternal long-axis section of the heart shows asymmetric septal hypertrophy with endocardial fibrous plaque. (**b**) Close-up of **a**: note the whitish endocardial plaque and the anterior mitral valve leaflet thickening. (**c**) Histology of the friction lesion showing endocardial fibrous thickening (Heidenhain trichrome)

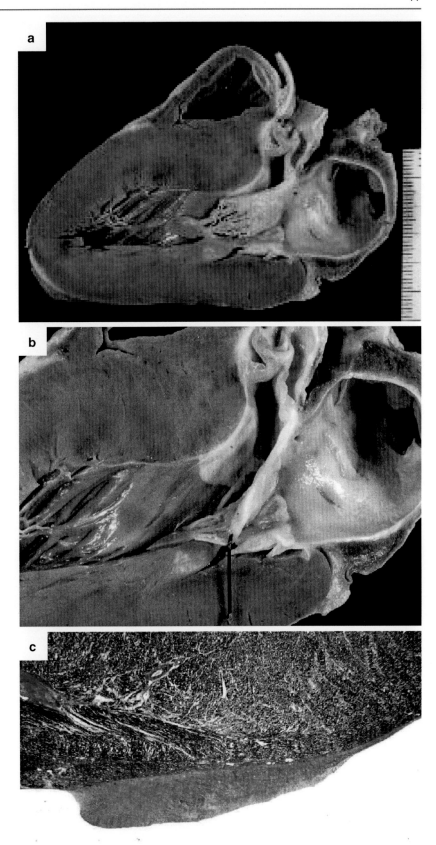

Fig. 4.3 Arrhythmic sudden cardiac death at rest due to hypertrophic cardiomyopathy in a 23-year-old man, with previous syncopal episodes and an in vivo diagnosis. (**a**) Parasternal long-axis section of the heart shows asymmetric septal hypertrophy (septal thickness about 30 mm) with endocardial fibrous plaque. (**b**) Short-axis view of the heart, showing massive left ventricular hypertrophy, with multiple whitish septal scars

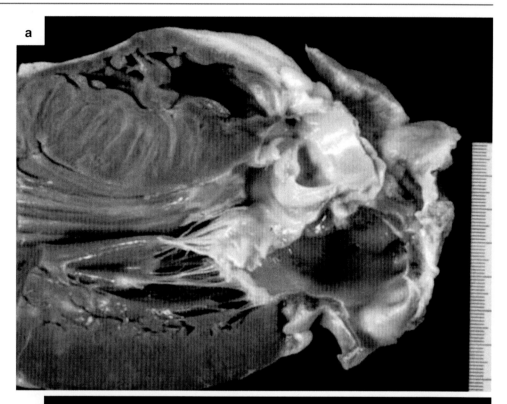

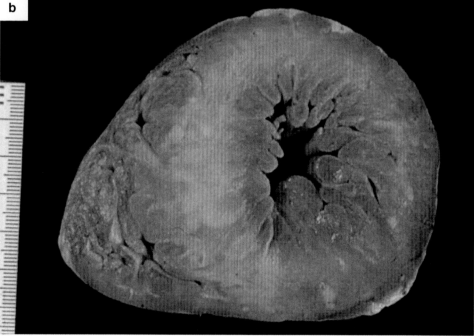

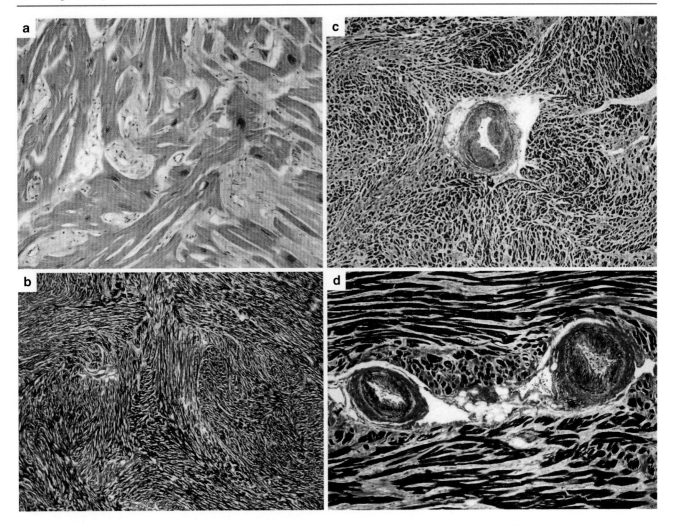

Fig. 4.4 Histological features of hypertrophic cardiomyopathy in sudden cardiac death victims. (**a**) Cardiac muscle cell disorganization (disarray), (hematoxylin–eosin). (**b**) Widespread fascicular myocardial disarray and interstitial fibrosis (Heidenhain trichrome). (**c, d**) Intramural small vessel disease (Heidenhain trichrome)

Fig. 4.5 Arrhythmic sudden cardiac death on effort due to hypertrophic cardiomyopathy in an 18-year-old soldier. (**a**) Cross section of the heart showing asymmetric septal hypertrophy and myocardial scars, (**b**) Parasternal long-axis section of the same. (**c**) Histology shows myocardial disarray, with replacement-type fibrosis (Heidenhain trichrome)

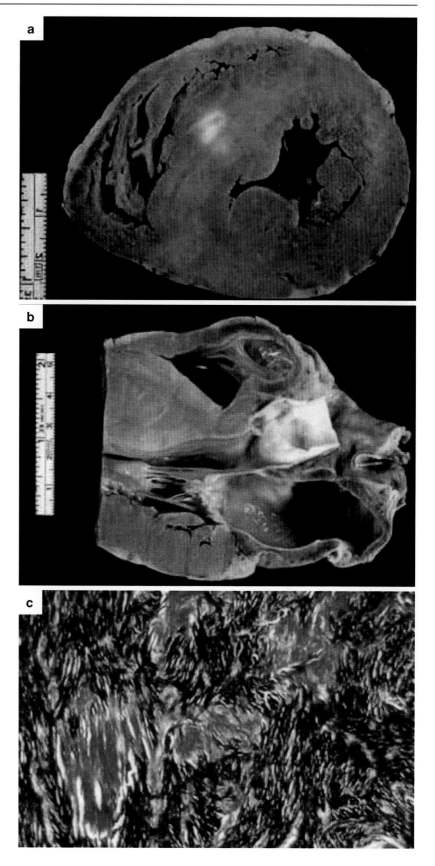

Fig. 4.6 Arrhythmic sudden cardiac death at rest due to hypertrophic cardiomyopathy in a 31-year-old man. (**a**) Parasternal longitudinal section of the heart showing asymmetric septal hypertrophy and myocardial scars. (**b**) Corresponding panoramic histological section showing multiple arcipelago-like areas of replacement-type fibrosis (Heidenhain trichrome)

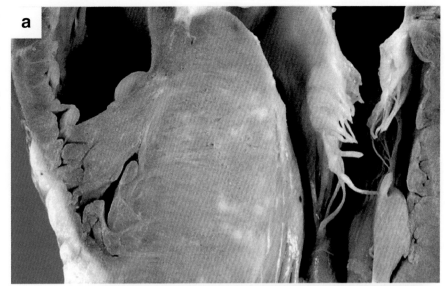

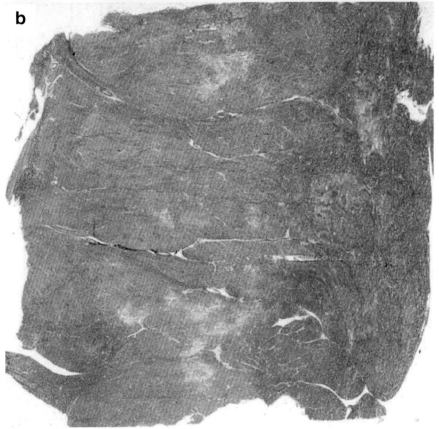

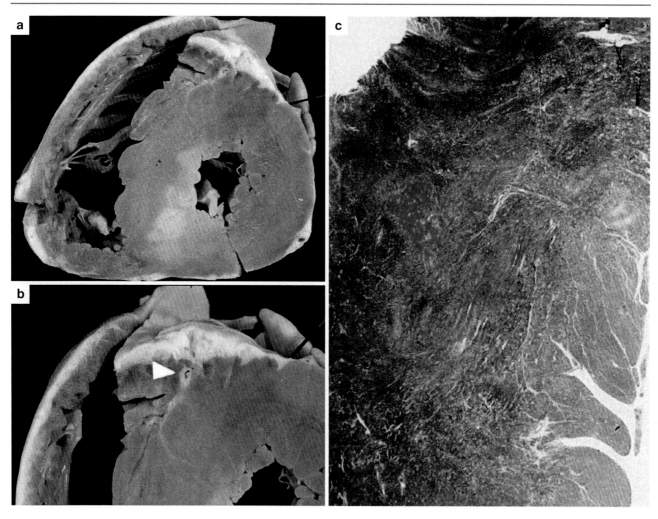

Fig. 4.7 Arrhythmic sudden cardiac death on effort due to hypertrophic cardiomyopathy in 15-year-old, previously asymptomatic boy, with a family history of the disease (father). (**a**) Short-axis view of the heart, showing massive concentric left ventricular hypertrophy and a large white scar in the posteroseptal area. (**b**) Intramyocardial course of the left anterior descending coronary artery (*arrowhead*). (**c**) Panoramic histological section of the septal area showing replacement-type fibrosis (Heidenhain trichrome)

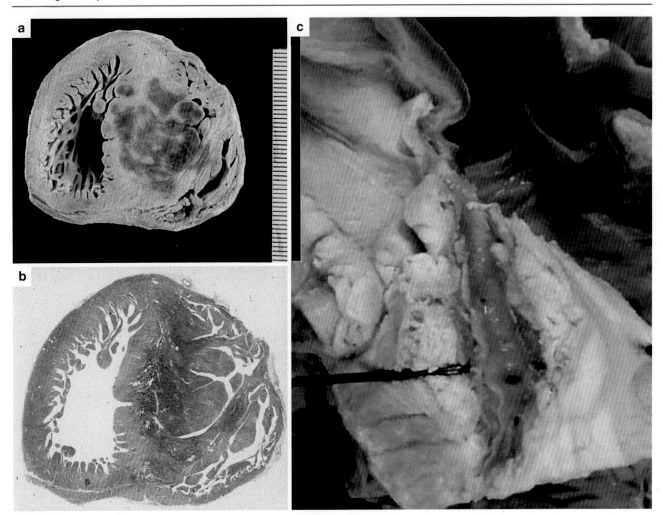

Fig. 4.8 Arrhythmic sudden cardiac death at school, due to hypertrophic cardiomyopathy in a 8-year-old asymptomatic boy. (**a**) Postmortem investigation reveales cardiomegaly with marked asymmetric septal hypertrophy (25-mm septal thickness vs. 7-mm thickness of the left ventricular free wall) and a hemorrhagic acute septal myocardial infarction. (**b**) Histological assessment revealed coagulation necrosis with interstitial hemorrhage as well as areas of replacement-type fibrosis (Heidenhain trichrome). (**c**) An intramural course of the left anterior descending coronary artery (2-mm-deep and 20-mm-long), corresponding to the region of the first and second septal branches, is visible

Fig. 4.9 Arrhythmic sudden cardiac death due to hypertrophic cardiomyopathy in a 29-year-old woman during jogging. (**a**) Transverse section of the heart specimen: note the absence of grossly visible fibrous scars and the deep intramural course of the left anterior descending coronary artery (*arrow*, depth 8 mm). (**b**) Marked myocyte disarray with tiny interstitial fibrosis (Heidenhain trichrome)

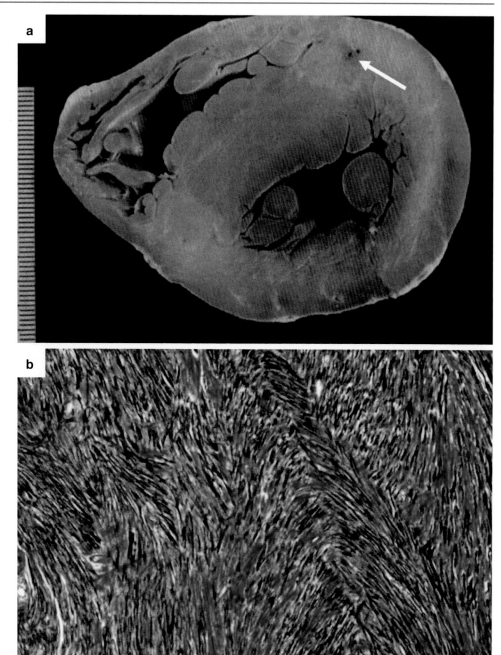

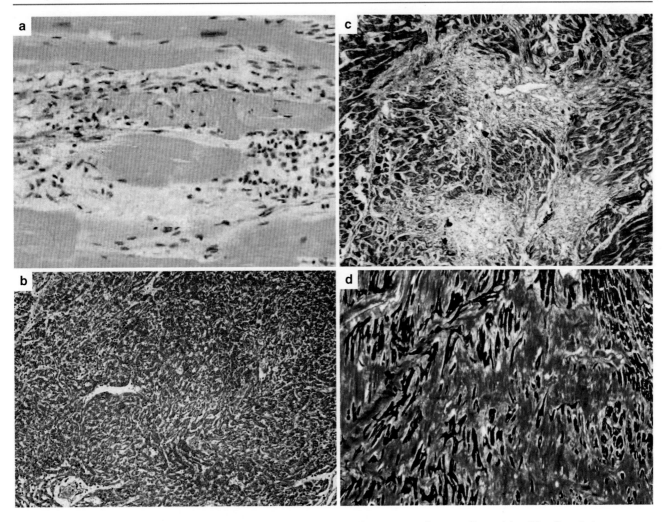

Fig. 4.10 Histological features of myocardial ischemic injury in young sudden cardiac death victims with hypertrophic cardiomyopathy and patent epicardial coronary arteries. (**a**) Cardiomyocyte necrosis, interstitial edema, and neutrophil diapedesis, close to hypertrophic cardiomyocytes (hematoxylin–eosin). (**b**) Coagulative myocyte necrosis (hematoxylin–eosin). (**c**) Subacute myocardial ischemia with myocytolysis and granulation tissue (Heidenhain trichrome). (**d**) Replacement-type fibrosis (scarring) (Heidenhain trichrome)

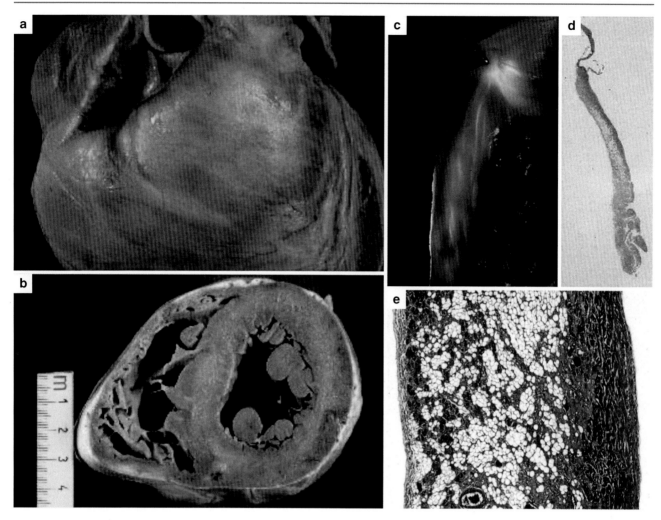

Fig. 4.11 Arrhythmic sudden cardiac death during exercise in a 26-year-old boy with arrhythmogenic cardiomyopathy (segmental form). (**a**) Gross view of the heart specimen showing a *yellow*, dilated pulmonary infundibulum. (**b**) Cross section of the heart with normal left ventricle and ventricular septum and a focal involvement of the poste- rior right ventricular free wall in the absence of wall thinning and aneu- rysm. (**c**) Gross view of the pulmonary infundibulum showing a very thin, translucent free wall. (**d**) Panoramic histological view of the pul- monary infundibulum showing fibrofatty replacement (Heidenhain tri- chrome). (**e**) Close-up of **d** (Heidenhain trichrome)

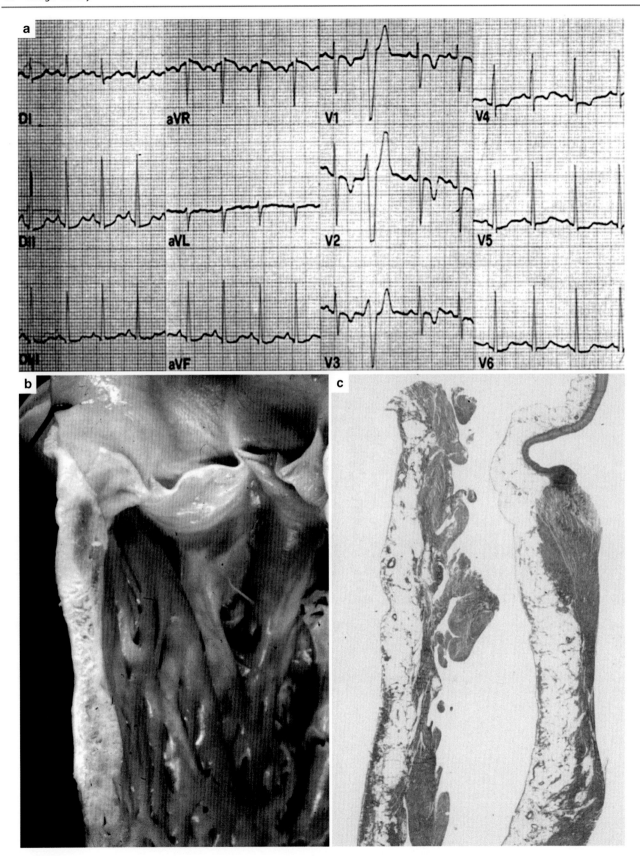

Fig. 4.12 Arrhythmic sudden cardiac death on effort in a 19-year-old boy with arrhythmogenic cardiomyopathy (segmental form). (**a**) Basal electrocardiogram showing inverted T wave in right precordial lead up to V4 and isolated premature ventricular beat with left bundle branch block morphology. (**b**) Gross examination of the right ventricular outflow tract shows a *yellow* appearance of the free wall, in the absence of wall thinning or aneurysm. (**c**) Panoramic, full thickness histological sections of the anterior and infundibular free walls showing transmural fibrofatty replacement with myocardium confined to the subendocardium (Heidenhain trichrome)

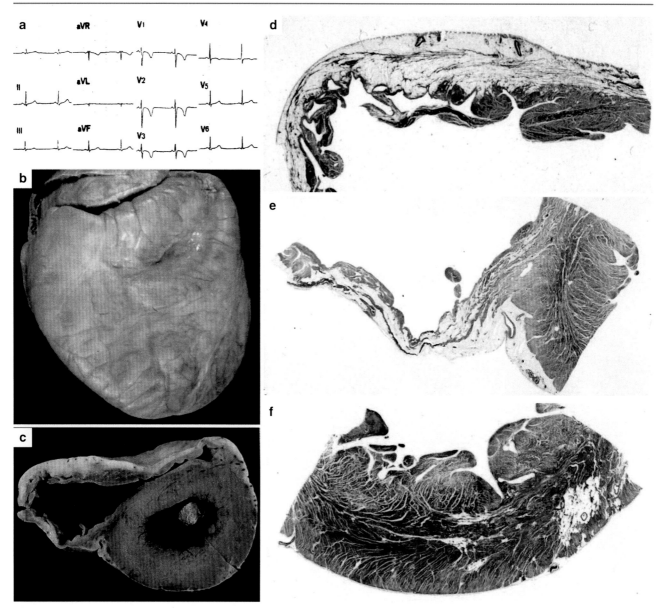

Fig. 4.13 Arrhythmic sudden cardiac death in a 17-year-old boy with arrhythmogenic cardiomyopathy, diffuse form. (**a**) Basal electrocardiogram showing inverted T wave in right precordial lead up to V4. (**b**) Gross view of the heart specimen showing a *yellow* appearance of the right ventricle and an aneurysm in the pulmonary outflow tract. (**c**) Through a mid-ventricular cross-section cut, aneurysms in the anterior and posterior right ventricular free walls and spotty involvement of the left ventricle are visible, with intact ventricular septum. (**d**, **e**) Histology of the anterior and posterior right ventricular free with remarkable, transmural fibrofatty replacement (Heidenhain trichrome). (**f**) Histology of the lateral left ventricular free with spotty, segmental fibrofatty replacement (Heidenhain trichrome)

Fig. 4.14 Arrhythmic sudden cardiac death in a 25-year-old boy with arrhythmogenic cardiomyopathy, diffuse form. (**a**) ECG tracing of ventricular fibrillation during cardiac arrest. (**b**) Gross examination of the heart specimen, four chamber section seen from behind: note the translucent anterior and infundibular wall. (**c**) Panoramic, full thickness histological section of the apical segment: transmural fibrofatty replacement of the right ventricle free wall is visible as compared to a normal left ventricular and septal myocardium (Heidenhain trichrome)

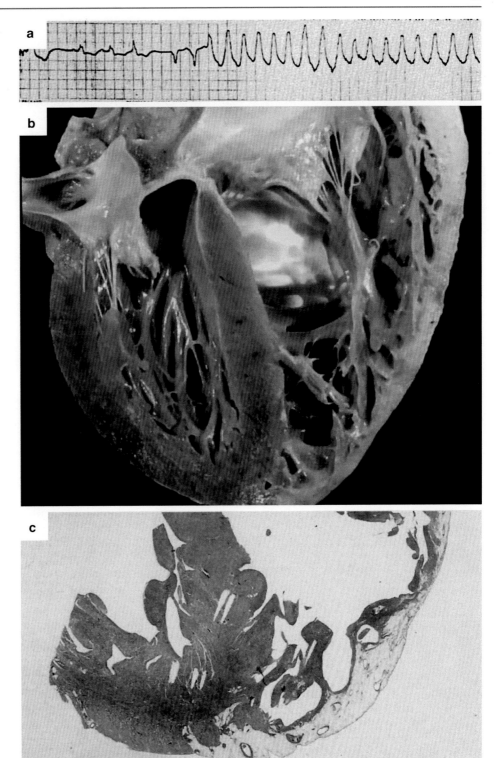

Fig. 4.15 Arrhythmic sudden cardiac death at rest in a 15-year-old boy, family member of an affected proband with arrhythmogenic cardiomyopathy and "healthy" carrier of a demoplakin mutation, (negative cardiological screening). (**a**) Cross section of the heart: there is no macroscopic evidence of fatty tissue infiltration nor aneurysms, whereas a gray band is evident in the subepicardial posterolateral region of the left ventricle. (**b**) Panoramic histological view of the posterior left ventricular wall showing a subepicardial band of acute–subacute myocyte necrosis with loose fibrous tissue and granulation tissue (Heidenhain trichrome). (**c**) Myocyte necrosis, myocytolysis, and polymorphous inflammatory infiltrates together with fibro-fatty repair are visible at higher magnification (hematoxylin–eosin)

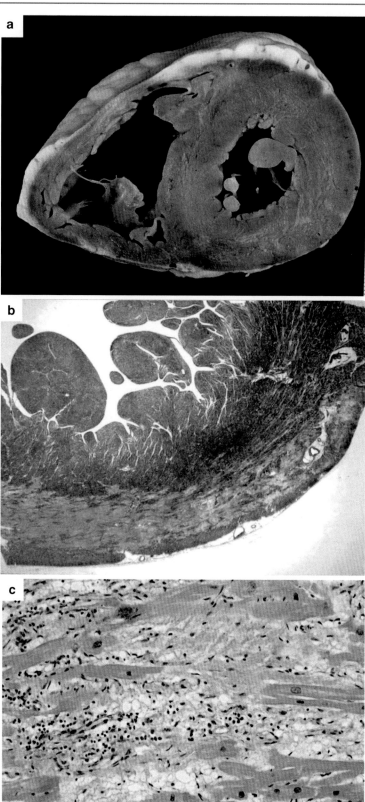

Fig. 4.16 Arrhythmic sudden cardiac death due to arrhythmogenic cardiomyopathy in a 39-year-old man with a family history of sudden death (two brothers). (**a**) Cross section of the heart showing pronounced fatty infiltration of the right ventricular free wall and normal ventricular septum: note the subepicardial involvement of the left ventricle. (**b**) Histological view of the right ventricular free wall showing transmural myocardial atrophy and remarkable fibrofatty replacement (Heidenhain trichrome). (**c**) Histological view of the left ventricular free wall showing fibrofatty replacement mostly confined to the subepicardium (Heidenhain trichrome)

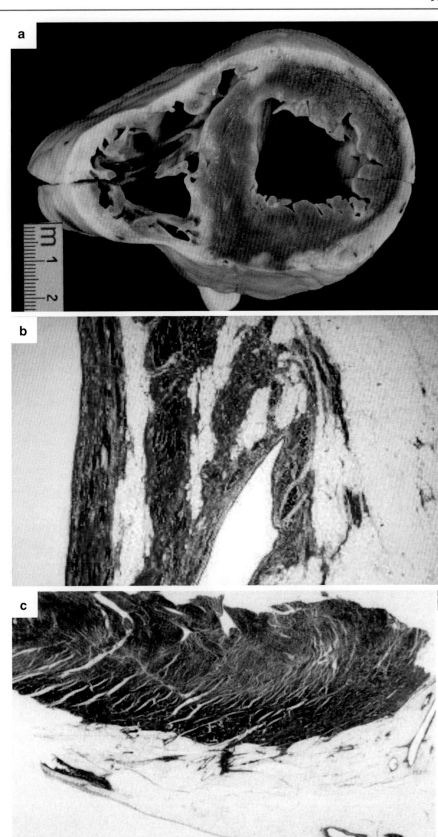

Fig. 4.17 Arrhythmic sudden cardiac death on effort, due to left dominant arrhythmogenic cardiomyopathy, in a 36-year-old man, previously asymptomatic. (**a**) Cross section of the heart specimen with normal appearance of right ventricular and septal myocardium but whitish appearance of the lateral left ventricular free wall, outer layer, with preserved wall thickness. (**b**) Panoramic histological section of the lateral left ventricular free wall shows subepicardial fibrofatty replacement (Heidenhain trichrome)

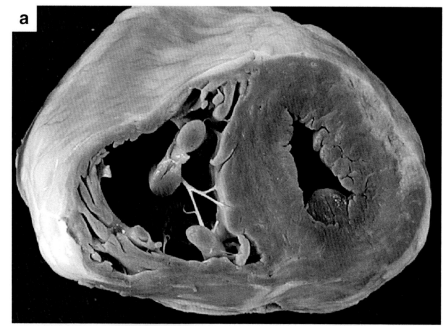

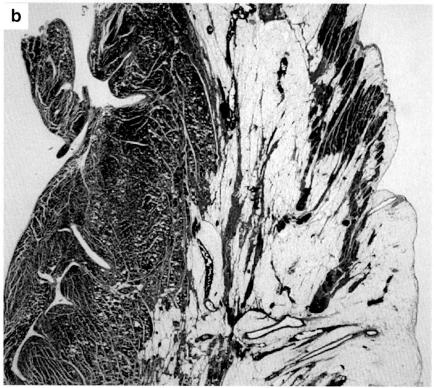

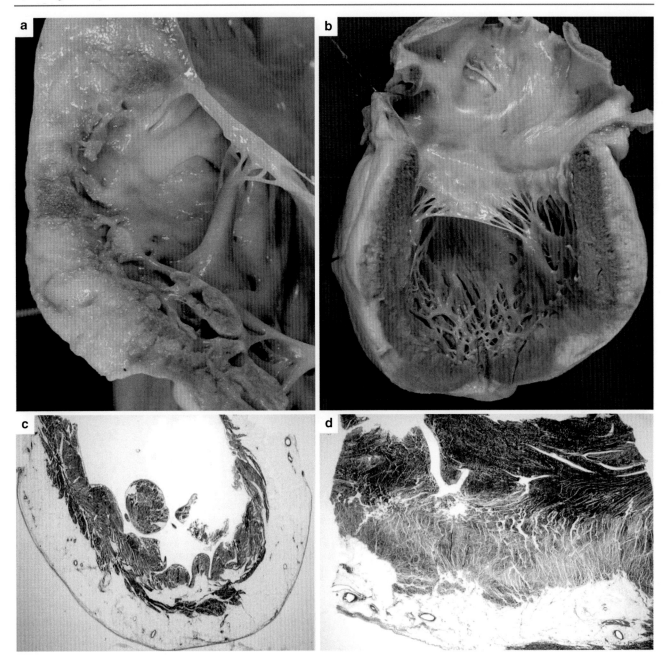

Fig. 4.18 Arrhythmic sudden cardiac death at rest due to arrhythmogenic cardiomyopathy in a 40-year-old man, previously asymptomatic. (**a**) View of the right ventricular inflow with lardaceous appearance of the lateral wall, subtricuspid aneurysm, and endocardial fibrous thickening. (**b**) View of the posterolateral left ventricular free wall: note the wave-front extension of fat from the epicardium toward the endocar-dium. (**c**) Panoramic histological section of the right ventricular free wall shows transmural fibrofatty replacement (Heidenhain trichrome). (**d**) Panoramic histological section of the left ventricular free wall with fibrofatty replacement in the outer subepicardial layer (Heidenhain trichrome)

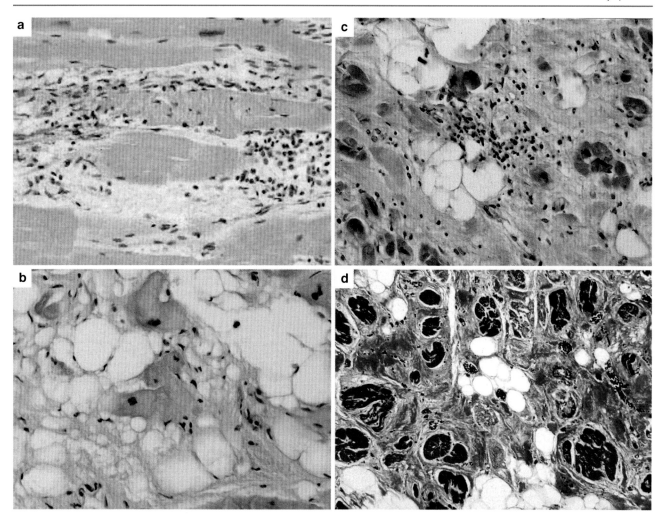

Fig. 4.19 From cell death to fibrofatty replacement in arrhythmogenic cardiomyopathy. (**a**) Histological features consistent with cardiomyocyte necrosis and inflammatory infiltrates in the early stages and during "pouseés" of disease progression (hematoxylin–eosin). (**b**) Adipocytes replacing dead and dying myocytes (hematoxylin-eosin). (**c**) Inflammatory infiltrates, mostly T lymphocytes and macrophages and early scarring associated with myocyte necrosis (hematoxylin–eosin). (**d**) Residual, surviving cardiomyocytes entrapped within fibrous and fatty tissue (Heidenhain trichrome)

References

1. Richardson P, McKenna WJ, Bristow M, Maisch B, Mautner B, O'Connell J, Olsen E, Thiene G, Goodwin J, Gyarfas I, Martin I, Nordet P. Report of the 1995 WHO/ISFC Task Force on the definition and classification of cardiomyopathies. Circulation. 1996;93:841–2.

2. Maron BJ, Towbin JA, Thiene G, Antzelevitch C, Corrado D, Arnett D, Moss AJ, Seidman CE, Young JB. Contemporary definitions and classification of the cardiomyopathies: an American Heart Association Scientific Statement from the Council on Clinical Cardiology, Heart Failure and Transplantation Committee; Quality of Care and Outcomes Research and Functional Genomics and Translational Biology Interdisciplinary Working Groups; and Council on Epidemiology and Prevention. Circulation. 2006;113:1807–16.

3. Elliott P, Andersson B, Arbustini E, Bilinska Z, Cecchi F, Charron P, Dubourg O, Kühl U, Maisch B, McKenna WJ, Monserrat L, Pankuweit S, Rapezzi C, Seferovic P, Tavazzi L, Keren A. Classification of the cardiomyopathies: a position statement from the European Society Of Cardiology Working Group on Myocardial and Pericardial Diseases. Eur Heart J. 2008;29:270–6.

4. Maron BJ, Shirani J, Poliac LC, Mathenge R, Roberts WC, Mueller FO. Sudden death in young competitive athletes. Clinical, demographic, and pathological profiles. JAMA. 1996;276:199–204.

5. Maron BJ, Roberts WJ, Epstein SE. Sudden death in hypertrophic cardiomyopathy: a profile of 78 patients. Circulation. 1982;65: 1388–94.

6. Maron BJ, Maron MS. Hypertrophic cardiomyopathy. Lancet. 2013;381:242–55.

7. Gersh BJ, Maron BJ, Bonow RO, Dearani JA, Fifer MA, Link MS, Naidu SS, Nishimura RA, Ommen SR, Rakowski H, Seidman CE, Towbin JA, Udelson JE, Yancy CW. 2011 ACCF/AHA guideline for the diagnosis and treatment of hypertrophic cardiomyopathy: executive summary: a report of the American College of Cardiology Foundation/American Heart Association Task Force on Practice Guidelines. Circulation. 2011;124:2761–96.

8. Elliott PM, Anastasakis A, Borger MA, Borggrefe M, Cecchi F, Charron P, Hagege AA, Lafont A, Limongelli G, Mahrholdt H, McKenna WJ, Mogensen J, Nihoyannopoulos P, Nistri S, Pieper PG, Pieske B, Rapezzi C, Rutten FH, Tillmanns C, Watkins H. 2014 ESC Guidelines on diagnosis and management of hypertrophic cardiomyopathy: the Task Force for the Diagnosis and Management of Hypertrophic Cardiomyopathy of the European Society of Cardiology (ESC). Eur Heart J. 2014;35:2733–79.

9. Teare D. Asymmetrical hypertrophy of the heart in young adults. Br Heart J. 1958;20:1–8.

10. Maron BJ, Roberts WC. Quantitative analysis of cardiac muscle cell disorganization in the ventricular septum of patients with hypertrophic cardiomyopathy. Circulation. 1979;59:689–706.

11. Maron BJ, Anan TJ, Roberts WC. Quantitative analysis of the distribution of cardiac muscle cell disorganization in the left ventricular wall of patients with hypertrophic cardiomyopathy. Circulation. 1981;63:882–94.

12. Maron BJ, Epstein SE, Roberts WC. Hypertrophic cardiomyopathy and transmural myocardial infarction without significant atherosclerosis of the extramural coronary arteries. Am J Cardiol. 1979;43:1086–102.

13. Maron BJ, Wolfson JK, Epstein SE, Roberts WC. Intramural ("small vessel") coronary artery disease in hypertrophic cardiomyopathy. J Am Coll Cardiol. 1986;8:545–57.

14. Varnava AM, Elliott PM, Sharma S, McKenna WJ, Davies MJ. Hypertrophic cardiomyopathy: the interrelation of disarray, fibrosis, and small vessel disease. Heart. 2000;84:476–82.

15. Basso C, Thiene G, Corrado D, Buja G, Melacini P, Nava A. Hypertrophic cardiomyopathy and sudden death in the young: pathologic evidence of myocardial ischemia. Hum Pathol. 2000;31:988–98.

16. Basso C, Thiene G, Mackey-Bojack S, Frigo AC, Corrado D, Maron BJ. Myocardial bridging, a frequent component of the hypertrophic cardiomyopathy phenotype, lacks systematic association with sudden cardiac death. Eur Heart J. 2009;30:1627–34.

17. Melacini P, Basso C, Angelini A, Calore C, Bobbo F, Tokajuk B, Bellini N, Smaniotto G, Zucchetto M, Iliceto S, Thiene G, Maron BJ. Clinicopathological profiles of progressive heart failure in hypertrophic cardiomyopathy. Eur Heart J. 2010;31:2111–23.

18. Chan RH, Maron BJ, Olivotto I, Pencina MJ, Assenza GE, Haas T, Lesser JR, Gruner C, Crean AM, Rakowski H, Udelson JE, Rowin E, Lombardi M, Cecchi F, Tomberli B, Spirito P, Formisano F, Biagini E, Rapezzi C, De Cecco CN, Autore C, Cook EF, Hong SN, Gibson CM, Manning WJ, Appelbaum E, Maron MS. Prognostic value of quantitative contrast-enhanced cardiovascular magnetic resonance for the evaluation of sudden death risk in patients with hypertrophic cardiomyopathy. Circulation. 2014;130:484–95.

19. Basso C, Burke M, Fornes P, Gallagher PJ, de Gouveia RH, Sheppard M, Thiene G, van der Wal A. Guidelines for autopsy investigation of sudden cardiac death. Virchows Arch. 2008;452:11–8.

20. de Noronha SV, Behr ER, Papadakis M, Ohta-Ogo K, Banya W, Wells J, Cox S, Cox A, Sharma S, Sheppard MN. The importance of specialist cardiac histopathological examination in the investigation of young sudden cardiac deaths. Europace. 2014;16:899–907.

21. Papadakis M, Raju H, Behr ER, De Noronha SV, Spath N, Kouloubinis A, Sheppard MN, Sharma S. Sudden cardiac death with autopsy findings of uncertain significance: potential for erroneous interpretation. Circ Arrhythm Electrophysiol. 2013;6:588–96.

22. Thiene G, Nava A, Corrado D, Rossi L, Pennelli N. Right ventricular cardiomyopathy and sudden death in young people. N Engl J Med. 1988;318:129–33.

23. Corrado D, Basso C, Pavei A, Michieli P, Schiavon M, Thiene G. Trends in sudden cardiovascular death in young competitive athletes after implementation of a preparticipation screening program. JAMA. 2006;296:1593–601.

24. Basso C, Corrado D, Marcus FI, Nava A, Thiene G. Arrhythmogenic right ventricular cardiomyopathy. Lancet. 2009;373:1289–300.

25. Basso C, Bauce B, Corrado D, Thiene G. Pathophysiology of arrhythmogenic cardiomyopathy. Nat Rev Cardiol. 2011;9: 223–33.

26. Thiene G. The research venture in arrhythmogenic right ventricular cardiomyopathy: a paradigm of translational medicine. Eur Heart J. 2015;36:837–46.

27. McKoy G, Protonotarios N, Crosby A, Tsatsopoulou A, Anastasakis A, Coonar A, Norman M, Baboonian C, Jeffrey S, McKenna WJ. Identification of a deletion in plakoglobin in arrhythmogenic right ventricular cardiomyopathy with palmoplantar keratoderma and wolly hair (Naxos disease). Lancet. 2000;355:2119–24.

28. Rampazzo A, Nava A, Malacrida S, Beffagna G, Bauce B, Rossi V, Zimbello R, Simionati B, Basso C, Thiene G, Towbin JA, Danieli GA. Mutation in human desmoplakin domain binding to plakoglobin causes a dominant form of arrhythmogenic right ventricular cardiomyopathy. Am J Hum Genet. 2002;71:1200–6.

29. Gerull B, Heuser A, Wichter T, Paul M, Basson CT, McDermott DA, Lerman BB, Markowitz SM, Ellinor PT, MacRae CA, Peters S, Grossmann KS, Michely B, Sasse-Klaassen S, Birchmeier W, Dietz R, Breithardt G, Schulze-Bahr E, Thierfelder L. Mutations in the desmosomal protein plakophilin-2 are common in arrhythmogenic right ventricular cardiomyopathy. Nat Genet. 2004;36:1162–4.

30. Pilichou K, Nava A, Basso C, Beffagna G, Bauce B, Lorenzon A, Frigo G, Vettori A, Valente M, Towbin J, Thiene G, Danieli GA, Rampazzo A. Mutations in desmoglein-2 gene are associated with arrhythmogenic right ventricular cardiomyopathy. Circulation. 2006;113:1171–9.

31. Basso C, Thiene G, Corrado D, Angelini A, Nava A, Valente M. Arrhythmogenic right ventricular cardiomyopathy: dysplasia, dystrophy, or myocarditis? Circulation. 1996;94:983–91.

32. Corrado D, Basso C, Thiene G, McKenna WJ, Davies MJ, Fontaliran F, Nava A, Silvestri F, Blomstrom-Lundqvist C, Wlodarska EK, Fontaine G, Camerini F. The spectrum of clinicopathologic manifestations of arrhythmogenic right ventricular cardiomyopathy/dysplasia. A Multicenter Study. J Am Coll Cardiol. 1997;30:1512–20.

33. Burke AP, Farb A, Tashko G, Virmani R. Arrhythmogenic right ventricular cardiomyopathy and fatty replacement of the right ventricular myocardium: are they different diseases? Circulation. 1998;97:1571–80.

34. Fornes P, Ratel S, Lecomte D. Pathology of arrhythmogenic right ventricular cardiomyopathy/dysplasia–an autopsy study of 20 forensic cases. J Forensic Sci. 1998;43:777–83.

35. Suárez-Mier MP, Aguilera B, Mosquera RM, Sánchez-de-León MS. Pathology of sudden death during recreational sports in Spain. Forensic Sci Int. 2013;226:188–96.

36. Lobo F, Silver MD, Butany J, Heggtviet HA. Left ventricular involvement in right ventricular dysplasia/cardiomyopathy. Can J Cardiol. 1999;15:1239–47.

37. Tavora F, Zhang M, Franco M, Oliveira JB, Li L, Fowler D, Zhao Z, Cresswell N, Burke A. Distribution of biventricular disease in arrhythmogenic cardiomyopathy: an autopsy study. Hum Pathol. 2012;43:592–6.

38. Basso C, Thiene G. Adipositas cordis, fatty infiltration of the right ventricle, and arrhythmogenic right ventricular cardiomyopathy. Just a matter of fat? Cardiovasc Pathol. 2005;14:37–41.

39. Marcus FI, Basso C, Gear K, Sorrell VL. Pitfalls in the diagnosis of arrhythmogenic right ventricular cardiomyopathy/dysplasia. Am J Cardiol. 2010;105:1036–9.

40. Basso C, Ronco F, Marcus F, Abudureheman A, Rizzo S, Frigo AC, Bauce B, Maddalena F, Nava A, Corrado D, Grigoletto F, Thiene G. Quantitative assessment of endomyocardial biopsy in arrhythmogenic right ventricular cardiomyopathy/dysplasia: an in vitro validation of diagnostic criteria. Eur Heart J. 2008;29:2760–71.

41. Marcus FI, McKenna WJ, Sherrill D, Basso C, Bauce B, Bluemke DA, Calkins H, Corrado D, Cox MG, Daubert JP, Fontaine G, Gear K, Hauer R, Nava A, Picard MH, Protonotarios N, Saffitz JE, Sanborn DM, Steinberg JS, Tandri H, Thiene G, Towbin JA, Tsatsopoulou A, Wichter T, Zareba W. Diagnosis of arrhythmogenic right ventricular cardiomyopathy/dysplasia: proposed modification of the Task Force Criteria. Circulation. 2010;121:1533–41.

42. Corrado D, Basso C, Leoni L, Tokajuk B, Bauce B, Frigo G, Tarantini G, Napodano M, Turrini P, Ramondo A, Daliento L, Nava A, Buja G, Iliceto S, Thiene G. Three-dimensional electroanatomic voltage mapping increases accuracy of diagnosing arrhythmogenic right ventricular cardiomyopathy/dysplasia. Circulation. 2005;111:3042–50.

43. Marra MP, Leoni L, Bauce B, Corbetti F, Zorzi A, Migliore F, Silvano M, Rigato I, Tona F, Tarantini G, Cacciavillani L, Basso C, Buja G, Thiene G, Iliceto S, Corrado D. Imaging study of ventricular scar in arrhythmogenic right ventricular cardiomyopathy: comparison of 3D standard electroanatomical voltage mapping and contrast-enhanced cardiac magnetic resonance. Circ Arrhythm Electrophysiol. 2012;5:91–100.

44. Pilichou K, Remme CA, Basso C, Campian ME, Rizzo S, Barnett P, Scicluna BP, Bauce B, van den Hoff MJ, de Bakker JM, Tan HL, Valente M, Nava A, Wilde AA, Moorman AF, Thiene G, Bezzina CR. Myocyte necrosis underlies progressive myocardial dystrophy in mouse dsg2-related arrhythmogenic right ventricular cardiomyopathy. J Exp Med. 2009;206:1787–802.

45. Valente M, Calabrese F, Angelini A, Basso C, Thiene G. In vivo evidence of apoptosis in arrhythmogenic right ventricular cardiomyopathy. Am J Pathol. 1998;152:479–84.

46. Syrris P, Ward D, Evans A, Asimaki A, Gandjbakhch E, Sen-Chowdhry S, McKenna WJ. Arrhythmogenic right ventricular dysplasia/cardiomyopathy associated with mutations in the desmosomal gene desmocollin-2. Am J Hum Genet. 2006;79: 978–84.

47. Beffagna G, De Bortoli M, Nava A, Salamon M, Lorenzon A, Zaccolo M, Mancuso L, Sigalotti L, Bauce B, Occhi G, Basso C, Lanfranchi G, Towbin JA, Thiene G, Danieli GA, Rampazzo A. Missense mutations in desmocollin-2 N-terminus, associated with arrhythmogenic right ventricular cardiomyopathy, affect intracellular localization of desmocollin-2 in vitro. BMC Med Genet. 2007;8:65.

48. Basso C, Czarnowska E, Della Barbera M, Bauce B, Beffagna G, Wlodarska EK, Pilichou K, Ramondo A, Lorenzon A, Wozniek O, Corrado D, Daliento L, Danieli GA, Valente M, Nava A, Thiene G, Rampazzo A. Ultrastructural evidence of intercalated disc remodelling in arrhythmogenic right ventricular cardiomyopathy: an electron microscopy investigation on endomyocardial biopsies. Eur Heart J. 2006;27:1847–54.

49. Rizzo S, Lodder EM, Verkerk AO, Wolswinkel R, Beekman L, Pilichou K, Basso C, Remme CA, Thiene G, Bezzina CR. Intercalated disc abnormalities, reduced Na+current density, and conduction slowing in desmoglein-2 mutant mice prior to cardiomyopathic changes. Cardiovasc Res. 2012;95:409–18.

50. Nava A, Bauce B, Basso C, Muriago M, Ramazzo A, Villanova C, Daliento L, Buja G, Corrado D, Danieli GA, Thiene G. Clinical profile and long term follow-up of 37 families with arrhythmogenic right ventricular cardiomyopathy. J Am Coll Cardiol. 2000;36: 2226–33.

51. Basso C, Corrado D, Bauce B, Thiene G. Arrhythmogenic right ventricular cardiomyopathy. Circ Arrhythm Electrophysiol. 2012;5: 1233–46.

52. Thiene G, Corrado D, Nava A, Rossi L, Poletti A, Boffa GM, Daliento L, Pennelli N. Right ventricular cardiomyopathy: is there evidence of an inflammatory aetiology? Eur Heart J. 1991;12: 22–25.

5

Myocarditis

Acute inflammation of the myocardium is another major cause of SCD in the young, particularly in children and adolescents [1–13]. The mechanism is mostly arrhythmic, since the affected young usually die without previous signs or symptoms and often during exercise performance.

At autopsy, the heart does not necessarily show ventricular dilatation and may appear grossly normal [7, 8, 13] (Fig. 5.1). At histology of the ventricular myocardium, patchy, either focal or diffuse, inflammatory infiltrates, together with interstitial edema and myocyte necrosis, may be found (Figs. 5.2–5.4). This pattern is quite different from that of fulminant myocarditis, associated with acute ventricular decompensation, pump failure, and cardiogenic shock, in which massive inflammatory infiltrates and cardiomyocyte necrosis are present. The inflammatory infiltrate usually consists of lymphocytes or may be polymorphic, with lymphocytes mixed to neutrophils/eosinophils [13, 14]. Immunostaining is essential for inflammatory cells characterization and is of help in patchy, focal forms (Fig. 5.5). This mild myocardial inflammation is enough to dysregulate the electrical order of the heart, enhancing the ectopic automatic mechanism of impulse onset. Release of cytokines, with interstitial edema and focal, patchy necrosis, may jeopardize the depolarization–repolarization phases of the myocardium, thus favoring triggered activity. In the subacute-chronic stages of myocarditis, varying degrees of replacement-type fibrosis might also account for electrical instability, with or without persistent inflammation (healing or healed myocarditis) (Fig. 5.6).

Among the various causes of myocarditis (infections, allergens, drugs, toxic agents, autoimmune reaction), viral infection is the most frequent etiology in SCD cases [7, 14–17].

Employment of PCR techniques, even in paraffin-embedded tissue, allows the identification of the causative infective agent [7, 14, 16]. In our experience (unpublished data), PCR was virus positive in 60 % of cases, with enterovirus ranking first, thus confirming the cardio-tropism and malignant behavior of coxsackievirus myocardial infection,

also in terms of arrhythmic risk. However, a large spectrum of viruses can be found at molecular autopsy, including DNA viruses like adenoviruses. The mechanism of myocardial injury by coxsackievirus consists of the release of a protease (2A), which cleaves dystrophin and collapses the cytoskeleton. By the way, coxsackievirus B and adenovirus share the same receptor (CAR) in the myocyte membrane [18, 19].

Exceptional nonviral causes of infective myocarditis have been also reported such as chlamydia pneumonia [20, 21], Whipple disease [22, 23], or tuberculosis [24]. Clinical presentation of myocarditis may be various (angina/myocardial "infarction" like, cardiogenic shock, arrhythmias), and endomyocardial biopsy is indicated as gold standard for diagnosis [14, 15, 25–27]. Of course, the study of myocardial samples should include molecular investigation to establish a causative viral agent.

The reported prevalence of myocarditis in SCD series varies from 2 to 42 %, questioning the diagnostic criteria employed at histology [7, 16]. Rare lymphocytes ($<7/mm^2$) in the myocardial interstitial space are a normal finding and by no way should be interpreted as a sign of myocarditis. We wonder how many cases of ion channel disease, as the true cause of SCD in the setting of a normal heart, have been misinterpreted as myocarditis [28, 29]. In a patient with arrhythmic presentation and myocarditis diagnosed by endomyocardial biopsy, an electrical storm may be pending so that temporary implantation of jacket defibrillator is indicated until resolution [15]. Respiratory or gastroenteric infections are quite common and may be that mild involvement of the myocardium occurs much more frequently than usually believed. Avoiding effort during fever of any infective origin is advisable.

SCD is rarely the clinical manifestation of giant cell myocarditis, which rather presents with cardiogenic shock [15]. On the opposite, cardiac sarcoidosis, either isolated or in the context of systemic disease, can be a cause of life-threatening ventricular arrhythmias and SCD even as first disease

© Springer-Verlag Milan 2016
G. Thiene et al., *Sudden Cardiac Death in the Young and Athletes: Text Atlas of Pathology and Clinical Correlates*,
DOI 10.1007/978-88-470-5776-0_5

manifestation [30–32], as to mimic arrhythmogenic cardio-myopathy [33] (Fig. 5.7).

Last but not least, toxicologic investigation is mandatory, to rule out unnatural causes, particularly in young adults and competitive athletes. For instance, myocarditis is a well-known cocaine-related cardiovascular complication [34–36]. It is mostly referred to as transient toxic cardiomyopathy, similar to catecholamine cardiomyopathy of pheochromocy-toma. Excess catecholamines leading to myocyte damage, due to calcium overload or transient coronary vasoconstric-tion with ischemic injury, are possible pathophysiologic mechanisms. It is still a matter of debate whether inflamma-tory infiltrates are a secondary reaction to myocyte death or whether they represent a primary hypersensitivity reaction to cocaine. Eosinophilic infiltrates usually suggest allergic dia-thesis or reaction to drug therapy (Fig. 5.8). While cocaine cardiotoxicity is often a cause of hypersensitivity myocardi-tis, anabolic androgenic steroids mostly accounting for lym-phocytic myocarditis and dilated cardiomyopathy [37] (Fig. 5.9).

5.1   Image Gallery

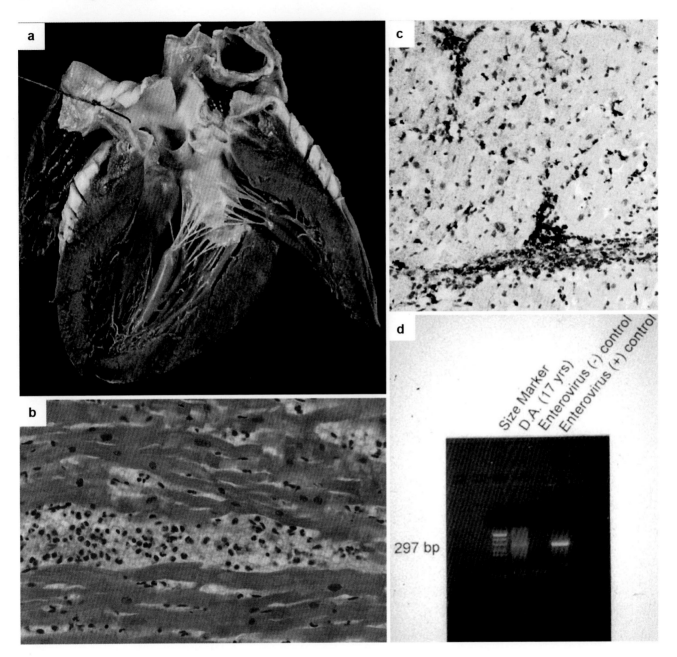

Fig. 5.1 Arrhythmic sudden cardiac death due to viral lymphocytic myocarditis in a 17-year-old boy who had a gastrointestinal flu 1 week before. (**a**) Grossly normal heart at autopsy. (**b**) Diffuse inflammatory cell infiltrates associated with interstitial edema and myocyte necrosis (hematoxylin–eosin). (**c**) At immunohistochemistry, the inflammatory infiltrate is rich in T lymphocytes (CD43 immunostaining). (**d**) PCR-proven acute myocarditis due to enterovirus infection

Fig. 5.2 Arrhythmic sudden cardiac death due to polymorphous myocarditis in a 9-year-old boy on effort. (**a**) Cross section of the heart with some subendocardial ischemia–reperfusion injury following cardiac arrest. (**b**) Diffuse inflammatory cell infiltrates associated with interstitial edema and myocyte necrosis (hematoxylin–eosin). (**c**) At higher magnification, polymorphous inflammatory cells including neutrophils and eosinophils (hematoxylin–eosin)

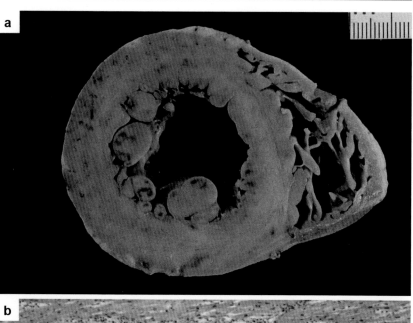

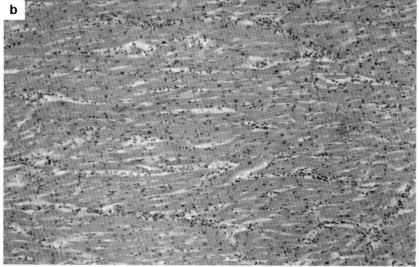

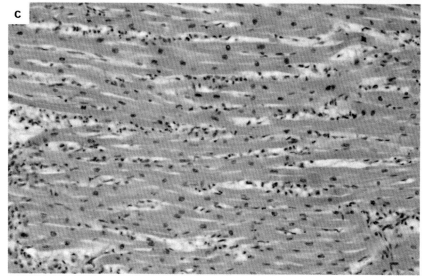

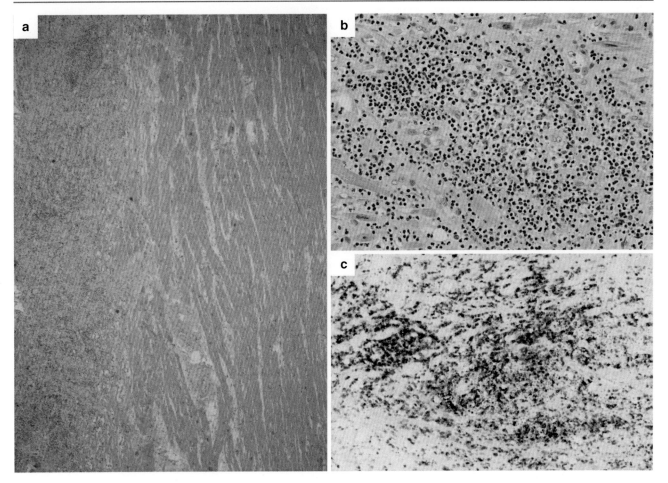

Fig. 5.3 Arrhythmic sudden cardiac death on effort due to lymphocytic myocarditis in a 22-year-old basketball player athlete. (**a**) Panoramic histology of the left ventricle: note the interstitial edema and massive inflammatory infiltrates in the outer layer of the left ventricular free wall (hematoxylin–eosin). (**b**) At higher magnification, diffuse polymorphous cell inflammatory infiltrates associated with myocyte necrosis (hematoxylin–eosin). (**c**) At immunohistochemistry, abundant T lymphocytes are seen (CD3 immunostaining)

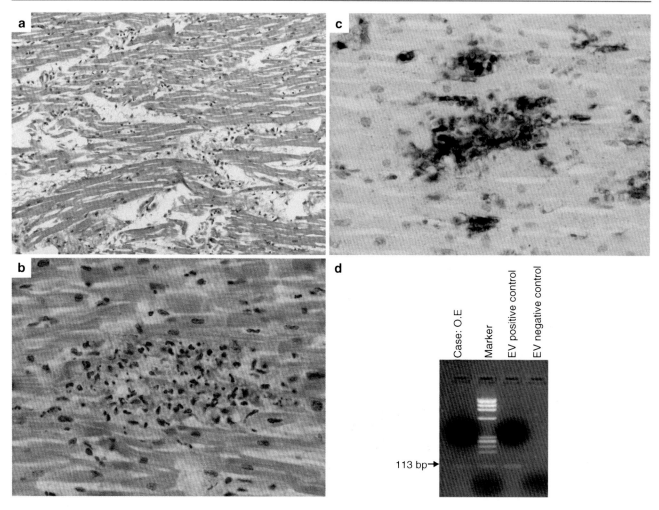

Fig. 5.4 Arrhythmic sudden cardiac death due to viral lymphocytic myocarditis in a 6-year-old girl with a history of flu 5 days preceding cardiac arrest. (**a**) Diffuse interstitial edema and inflammatory infiltrates (hematoxylin–eosin). (**b**) At higher magnification, focus of inflammatory infiltrate associated with myocyte necrosis (hematoxylin–eosin). (**c**) At immunohistochemistry, the inflammatory infiltrate is rich in T lymphocytes (CD3 immunostaining). (**d**) PCR-proven lymphocytic myocarditis due to enterovirus infection

Fig. 5.5 Arrhythmic sudden cardiac death due to patchy lymphocytic myocarditis in a 25-year-old man at rest with a grossly normal heart. (**a**) Scattered inflammatory infiltrates (mononuclear cells) are visible in the myocardium (hematoxylin–eosin). (**b**) At immunohistochemistry, T lymphocytes are evident in the interstitium (CD3 immunostaining)

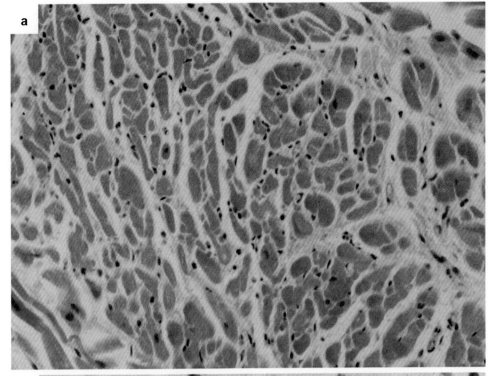

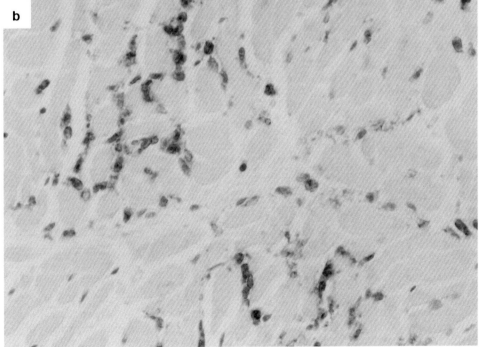

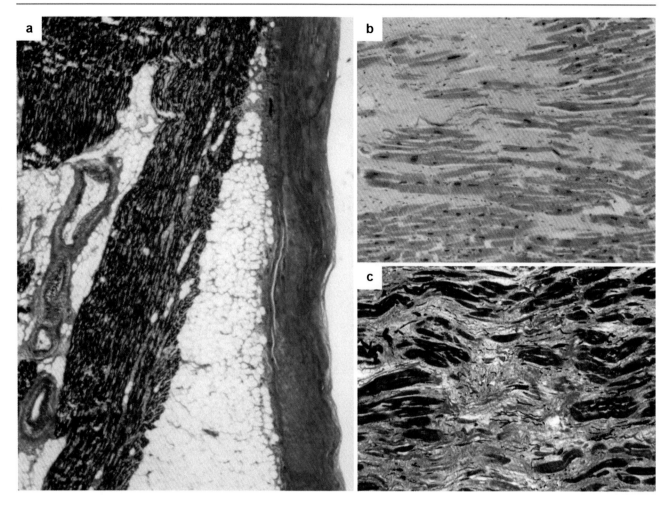

Fig. 5.6 Arrhythmic sudden cardiac death in a 26-year-old man on effort due to healed myopericarditis. (a) Histology of the right ventricular free wall: note the thickened, fibrotic pericardium (Heidenhain trichrome). (b) At higher magnification, histology of both the right and left ventricular myocardium shows patchy areas of replacement-type fibrosis (hematoxylin–eosin). (c) Other field with patchy fibrosis (Heidenhain trichrome)

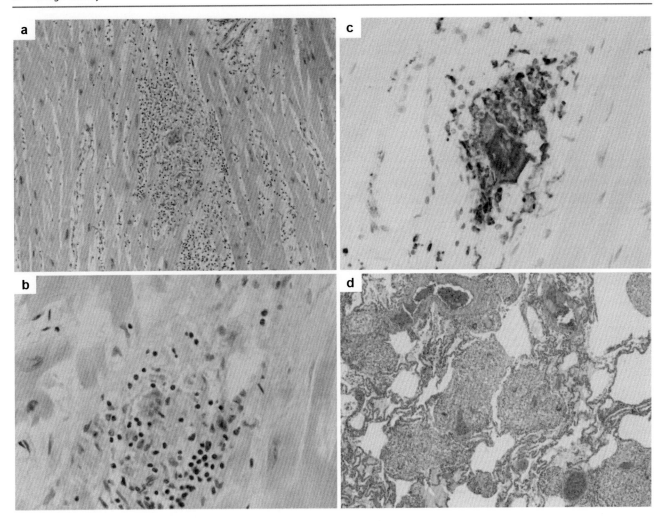

Fig. 5.7 Arrhythmic sudden cardiac death due to sarcoid myocarditis in a 32-year-old man at rest. (**a**) At histology of the myocardium, fibrosis and noncaseating granulomas are visible, consisting of aggregates of epithelioid histiocytes with minimal inflammation and large multinucleated giant cells (hematoxylin–eosin). (**b**) Close-up of A (hematoxylin–eosin). (**c**) At immunohistochemistry, the multinucleated giant cells are positive for macrophage marker (CD68 immunostaining). (**d**) At histology, the lungs also present with noncaseating granulomas (hematoxylin–eosin)

Fig. 5.8 Arrhythmic sudden
cardiac death due to
eosinophilic myocarditis in a
25-year-old bodybuilder
while sleeping, with a history
of anabolic androgenic
steroids abuse.
(**a**) Interstitial edema
and inflammatory infiltrates
rich in eosinophilis
(hematoxylin–eosin).
(**b**) Close-up of **a**
(hematoxylin–eosin)

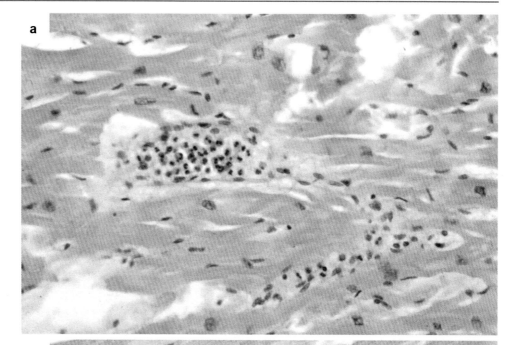

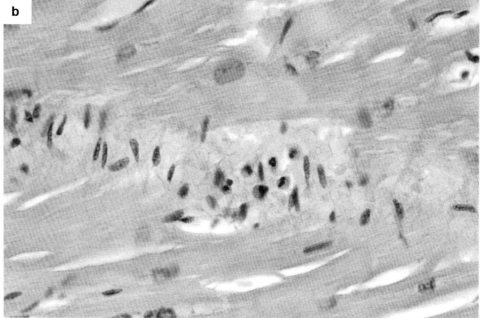

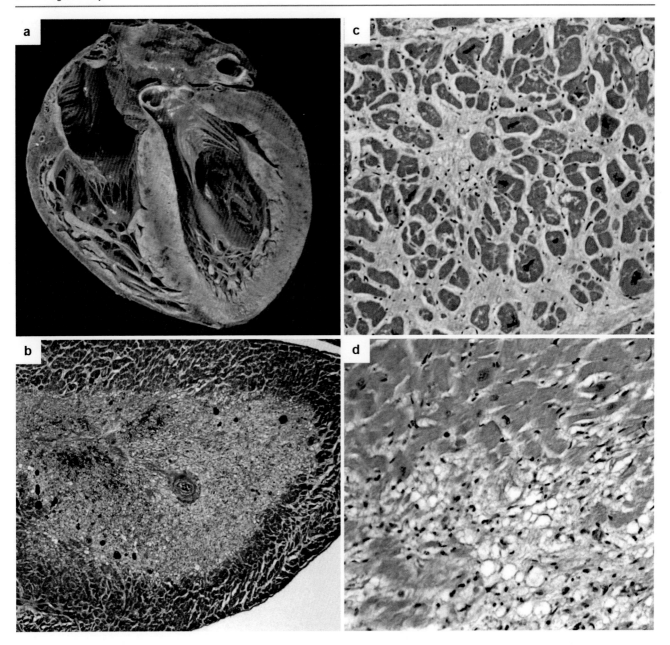

Fig. 5.9 Heart failure death following aborted arrhythmic sudden cardiac death during training due to healing myocarditis evolving into dilated cardiomyopathy in a 31-year-old bodybuilder with anabolic androgenic steroids abuse. (**a**) Cardiomegaly (weight 900 g) with biventricular eccentric hypertrophy. (**b**) Myocytolysis in the subendo- cardial trabeculae (Heidenhain trichrome). (**c**) Hypertrophic myocytes with dysmetric and dysmorphic nuclei, interstitial and replacement- type fibrosis, and rare inflammatory infiltrates (hematoxylin–eosin). (**d**) At higher magnification, myocytolysis (hematoxylin–eosin)

References

1. Topaz O, Edwards JE. Pathologic features of sudden death in children, adolescents, and young adults. Chest. 1985;87:476–82.
2. Driscoll DJ, Edwards WD. Sudden unexpected death in children and adolescents. J Am Coll Cardiol. 1985;5(6 Suppl):118B–21.
3. Phillips M, Robinowitz M, Higgins JR, Boran KJ, Reed T, Virmani R. Sudden cardiac death in Air Force recruits. JAMA. 1986;256:2696–9.
4. Haas JE. Myocarditis and sudden, unexpected death in childhood. Pediatr Pathol. 1988;8:443–6.
5. Silka MJ, Kron J, Walance CG, Cutler JE, McAnulty JH. Assessment and follow-up of pediatric survivors of sudden cardiac death. Circulation. 1990;82:341–9.
6. Shen WK, Edwards WD, Hammill SC, Bailey KR, Ballard DJ, Gersh BJ. Sudden unexpected nontraumatic death in 54 young adults: a 30-year population-based study. Am J Cardiol. 1995;76:148–52.
7. Basso C, Calabrese F, Corrado D, Thiene G. Postmortem diagnosis in sudden cardiac death victims: macroscopic, microscopic and molecular findings. Cardiovasc Res. 2001;50:290–330.
8. Corrado D, Basso C, Thiene G. Sudden cardiac death in young people with apparently normal heart. Cardiovasc Res. 2001;50:399–408.
9. Theleman KP, Kuiper JJ, Roberts WC. Acute myocarditis (predominately lymphocytic) causing sudden death without heart failure. Am J Cardiol. 2001;88:1078–83.
10. Eckart RE, Scoville SL, Shry EA, Potter RN, Tedrow U. Causes of sudden death in young female military recruits. Am J Cardiol. 2006;97:1756–8.
11. Kitulwatte ID, Kim PJ, Pollanen MS. Sudden death related myocarditis: a study of 56 cases. Forensic Sci Med Pathol. 2010;6:13–9.
12. Larsson E, Wesslén L, Lindquist O, Baandrup U, Eriksson L, Olsen E, Rolf C, Friman G. Sudden unexpected cardiac deaths among young Swedish orienteers–morphological changes in hearts and other organs. APMIS. 1999;107:325–36.
13. Thiene G, Carturan E, Corrado D, Basso C. Prevention of sudden cardiac death in the young and in athletes: dream or reality? Cardiovasc Pathol. 2010;19:207–17.
14. Basso C, Calabrese F, Angelini A, Carturan E, Thiene G. Classification and histological, immunohistochemical, and molecular diagnosis of inflammatory myocardial disease. Heart Fail Rev. 2013;18:673–81.
15. Caforio AL, Pankuweit S, Arbustini E, Basso C, Gimeno-Blanes J, Felix SB, Fu M, Heliö T, Heymans S, Jahns R, Klingel K, Linhart A, Maisch B, McKenna W, Mogensen J, Pinto YM, Ristic A, Schultheiss HP, Seggewiss H, Tavazzi L, Thiene G, Yilmaz A, Charron P, Elliott PM. Current state of knowledge on aetiology, diagnosis, management, and therapy of myocarditis: a position statement of the European Society of Cardiology Working Group on Myocardial and Pericardial Diseases. Eur Heart J. 2013;34:2636–48.
16. Basso C, Burke M, Fornes P, Gallagher PJ, de Gouveia RH, Sheppard M, Thiene G, van der Wal A, Association for European Cardiovascular Pathology. Guidelines for autopsy investigation of sudden cardiac death. Virchows Arch. 2008;452:11–8.
17. Gaaloul I, Riabi S, Harrath R, Evans M, Salem NH, Mlayeh S, Huber S, Aouni M. Sudden unexpected death related to enterovirus myocarditis: histopathology, immunohistochemistry and molecular pathology diagnosis at post-mortem. BMC Infect Dis. 2012;12:212.
18. Tomko RP, Xu R, Philipson L. HCAR and MCAR: the human and mouse cellular receptors for subgroup C adenoviruses and group B coxsackieviruses. Proc Natl Acad Sci U S A. 1997;94:3352–6.
19. He Y, Chipman PR, Howitt J, Bator CM, Whitt MA, Baker TS, Kuhn RJ, Anderson CW, Freimuth P, Rossmann MG. Interaction of coxsackievirus B3 with the full length coxsackievirus-adenovirus receptor. Nat Struct Biol. 2001;8:874–8.
20. Wesslén L, Påhlson C, Lindquist O, Hjelm E, Gnarpe J, Larsson E, Baandrup U, Eriksson L, Fohlman J, Engstrand L, Linglöf T, Nyström-Rosander C, Gnarpe H, Magnius L, Rolf C, Friman G. An increase in sudden unexpected cardiac deaths among young Swedish orienteers during 1979–1992. Eur Heart J. 1996;17:902–10.
21. Wesslén L, Påhlson C, Friman G, Fohlman J, Lindquist O, Johansson C. Myocarditis caused by Chlamydia pneumoniae (TWAR) and sudden unexpected death in a Swedish elite orienteer. Lancet. 1992;340:427–8.
22. McGettigan P, Mooney EE, Sinnott M, Sweeney EC, Feely J. Sudden death in Whipple's disease. Postgrad Med J. 1997;73:509–11.
23. Mooney EE, Kenan DJ, Sweeney EC, Gaede JT. Myocarditis in Whipple's disease: an unsuspected cause of symptoms and sudden death. Mod Pathol. 1997;10:524–9.
24. Amonkar G, Rupani A, Shah V, Parmar H. Sudden death in tuberculous myocarditis. Cardiovasc Pathol. 2009;18:247–8.
25. Leone O, Veinot JP, Angelini A, Baandrup UT, Basso C, Berry G, Bruneval P, Burke M, Butany J, Calabrese F, d'Amati G, Edwards WD, Fallon JT, Fishbein MC, Gallagher PJ, Halushka MK, McManus B, Pucci A, Rodriguez ER, Saffitz JE, Sheppard MN, Steenbergen C, Stone JR, Tan C, Thiene G, van der Wal AC, Winters GL. 2011 consensus statement on endomyocardial biopsy from the Association for European Cardiovascular Pathology and the Society for Cardiovascular Pathology. Cardiovasc Pathol. 2012;21:245–74.
26. Frustaci A, Bellocci F, Olsen EGJ. Results of biventricular endomyocardial biopsy in survivors of cardiac arrest with apparently normal hearts. Am J Cardiol. 1994;74:890–5.
27. Thiene G, Bruneval P, Veinot J, Leone O. Diagnostic use of the endomyocardial biopsy: a consensus statement. Virchows Arch. 2013;463:1–5.
28. Zhang M, Tavora F, Zhang Y, Ripple M, Fowler D, Li L, Zhao Z, Burke A. The role of focal myocardial inflammation in sudden unexpected cardiac and non cardiac deaths–a clinic-opathological study. Int J Legal Med. 2013;127:131–8.
29. De Salvia A, De Leo D, Carturan E, Basso C. Sudden cardiac death, borderline myocarditis and molecular diagnosis: evidence or assumption? Med Sci Law. 2011;51(Suppl 1):S27–9.
30. James TN. Clinicopathologic correlations. De subitaneis mortibus. XXV. Sarcoid heart disease. Circulation. 1977;56:320–6.
31. Tavora F, Cresswell N, Li L, Ripple M, Solomon C, Burke A. Comparison of necropsy findings in patients with sarcoidosis dying suddenly from cardiac sarcoidosis versus dying suddenly from other causes. Am J Cardiol. 2009;104:571–7.
32. Bagwan IN, Hooper LV, Sheppard MN. Cardiac sarcoidosis and sudden death. The heart may look normal or mimic other cardiomyopathies. Virchows Arch. 2011;458:671–8.
33. Vasaiwala SC, Finn C, Delpriore J, Leya F, Gagermeier J, Akar JG, Santucci P, Dajani K, Bova D, Picken MM, Basso C, Marcus F, Wilber DJ. Prospective study of cardiac sarcoid mimicking arrhythmogenic right ventricular dysplasia. J Cardiovasc Electrophysiol. 2009;20:473–6.
34. Karch SB, Billingham ME. The pathology and etiology of cocaine-induced heart disease. Arch Pathol Lab Med. 1988;112:225–30.
35. Virmani R, Robinowitz M, Smialek JE, Smyth DF. Cardiovascular effects of cocaine: an autopsy study of 40 patients. Am Heart J. 1988;115:1068–76.
36. Pilgrim JL, Woodford N, Drummer OH. Cocaine in sudden and unexpected death: a review of 49 post-mortem cases. Forensic Sci Int. 2013;227:52–9.
37. Montisci M, El Mazloum R, Cecchetto G, Terranova C, Ferrara SD, Thiene G, Basso C. Anabolic androgenic steroids abuse and cardiac death in athletes: morphological and toxicological findings in four fatal cases. Forensic Sci Int. 2012;217:e13–8.

Valve Disease

6

6.1 Aortic Valve

6.1.1 Aortic Valve Stenosis

SCD may occur in young people affected by congenital aortic valve stenosis, whether unicuspid or bicuspid with dysplastic cusps [1, 2] (Figs. 6.1, and 6.2). At a young age, the cusps rarely present with a dystrophic calcification, a phenomenon which usually occurs in adult or in the elderly [3–5]. When it happens prematurely, it is usually secondary to endocarditis (Fig. 6.3). SCD is arrhythmic and the arrhythmogenic substrate consists of left ventricular hypertrophy and subendocardial ischemia, in terms of myocytolysis and replacement-type fibrosis (Fig. 6.3) [1, 6].

Subendocardial fibrotic scars are a frequent observation in patients with aortic valve stenosis dying suddenly. The injury is ischemic in nature, since vacuolization of cardiomyocytes and even acute coagulation necrosis are also observed (Fig. 6.3). Clearly, a discrepancy between blood flow demand, due to compensatory left ventricular hypertrophy as a consequence of severe trans-valvular gradient and pressure overload, and coronary artery blood perfusion precipitates ischemic damage, even in the absence of coronary artery disease. An impairment of coronary reserve due to wall stiffness, with constriction of coronary microvasculature during diastole, is an additional factor.

6.1.2 Bicuspid Aortic Valve

A normally functioning bicuspid aortic valve can at risk of SCD. The cardiac arrest is the consequence of spontaneous rupture of the ascending aorta due to dissection, hemopericardium, and cardiac tamponade, because of coexistent aortopathy [1].

The occurrence of aortic dissection in bicuspid aortic valve is five- to sevenfold than the one occurring in normal population with tricuspid aortic valve and nearly 5–6 % of

people with aortic dissection show a bicuspid aortic valve. This suggests that bicuspid valve "per se" is a risk factor of aortic dissection, as it is in Marfan syndrome [7, 8].

When bicuspid aortic valve is associated with isthmic aortic coarctation (40–50 % of patients with coarctation present a bicuspid aortic valve), a plausible explanation for the aortic dissection might be the severe hypertension in the prestenotic ascending aorta (Fig. 6.4). However, this is not the case of the dissection occurring in isolated bicuspid aortic valve (Figs. 6.5, and 6.6). A severe disruption of the tunica media, with elastic fragmentation, medial necrosis with loss of smooth muscle cells, and mucoid substance accumulation, is a regular finding at histology [1]. The picture is similar to that observed in Marfan syndrome, the natural history of which is notoriously characterized by early spontaneous aortic dissection by the age of 30–40 years (Figs. 6.7, and 6.8) (see also Chap. 3).

The weakness of tunica media is associated with dilatation of the ascending aorta, which starts prematurely by 15–20 years and then progresses with time up to 4–5 cm in diameter in association with aortic valve incompetence. Aortic dimension of 4.5–5.0 cm is considered the threshold for surgical replacement of the ascending aorta, but we have observed cases of bicuspid aortic valve, aortic dissection, and SCD with much less dilatation.

The atrophy of the elastic fibers of the tunica media accounts for stiffness of the aortic wall with scarce systolic–diastolic excursion, a phenomenon easily detectable at echo and clearly indicating an elastic impairment [9, 10].

The association of bicuspid aortic valve and a degenerative pathology of the aortic root suggest the possible existence of a "bicuspid aortic valve syndrome" in which the bicuspid aortic valve is just one congenital defect in the setting of a developmental pathology of the entire aortic root. Maldevelopment of neural crest, which plays a role in the embryology of both the semilunar valves and the ascending aorta–aortic arch, has been advanced as etiopathogenetic factor.

© Springer-Verlag Milan 2016
G. Thiene et al., *Sudden Cardiac Death in the Young and Athletes: Text Atlas of Pathology and Clinical Correlates*,
DOI 10.1007/978-88-470-5776-0_6

6.1.3 Supravalvular Aortic Stenosis

It is an autosomal dominant disorder of the elastic fibers, due to deletion of elastin gene at the level of chromosome 7 [12–14]. The lesion is located on the ascending aorta with the shape of a diaphragm, hourglass, or diffuse hypoplasia [12, 13] (Fig. 6.9). It may be either isolated or associated with William's syndrome, with typical face and intellectual disorders.

The supravalvular stenosis is due to a localized or diffuse intimal fibrous plaque, as a consequence of ventricular systolic ejection on a rigid aorta due to the abnormally stiff elastic tunica media. The coronary ostia may be involved and obstructed.

Cases have been reported of associated anomalies of the aortic valve, the cusps of which may be thickened and fused with the aortic wall. In the latter case, the coronary ostium may be sequestered. In any case, the arrhythmogenic substrate accounting for arrhythmic SCD is an ischemic injury of the myocardium due to ventricular pressure overload, as it is in aortic valve stenosis.

6.2   Mitral Valve

6.2.1   Mitral Valve Prolapse

SCD occurring in young people affected by mitral valve prolapse is arrhythmic, not mechanical [15–17]. Certainly, rupture of chordae tendinae may complicate mitral valve prolapse during natural history and account for abrupt pulmonary edema, but it is rarely a cause of SCD.

In the young, we are dealing with a mitral valve prolapse with coarse deformation of the leaflets, which appear ballooning and thickened due to myxoid changes, in the absence of moderate to severe mitral incompetence and with apparently intact subvalvular apparatus, except for chordal elongation and thinning [17]. The posterior leaflet is usually involved, mostly the medial scallop, well outlined by hooding and mucoid thickening (Figs. 6.10, and 6.11). However, the anterior leaflet may also be affected.

SCD arrhythmic death can be preceded by life-threatening ventricular arrhythmias [17]. The ominous cardiac electrical instability, up to electrical turmoil and cardiac arrest, remains obscure. Several hypothesis have been postulated (endocardial friction of the chordae tendinae, concomitant fatty infiltration of the right ventricle, or specialized conduction system abnormalities), but they are not at all con-vincing to explain such an abrupt electrical disorder [18–26]. Previous pathology studies in mitral valve prolapse patients dying suddenly mostly focused on mitral valve structural alterations, suggesting a role for leaflets length and thickness, and presence and extent of endocardial plaques. Surprisingly, no investigation did systematically address the left ventricular myocardium to search for the substrate of electrical instability, except for few anecdotic cases. By a thorough histology of the left ventricle, we found evidence of patchy replacement-type fibrosis in the mitral valve papillary muscle as well as in the posterobasal free wall, with or without endocardial plaque, a finding which represents a much more plausible arrhythmogenic substrate, detectable in vivo by cardiac magnetic resonance [17] (Figs. 6.10, and 6.11). In other words, we are dealing with an arrhythmic disorder, which finds an explanation in a myocardial injury associated to mitral valve prolapse. In these circumstances, the term "arrhythmic mitral valve syndrome" is justifiable.

6.3   Tricuspid Valve

6.3.1   Ebstein's Anomaly

It is well known that patients with Ebstein's anomaly of the tricuspid valve may present arrhythmias, especially supraventricular tachycardia with ventricular preexcitation in the setting of Wolff–Parkinson–White syndrome [27–30]. The downward displacement of the septal leaflet of the tricuspid valve, which is pathognomonic of the disease, may be associated with accessory pathways (septal "Kent fascicles"), because of the AV ring maldevelopment and direct contact of the atrial with ventricular septal working myocardium, which represents the substrate for AV reentry with onset of supraventricular tachycardia.

There are minor forms of Ebstein's anomaly, associated with mild tricuspid valve dysfunction, with only minimal downward displacement of septal tricuspid leaflet (so-called microEbstein), but enough to delineate a clear contact between septal atria and ventricular myocardium, as to bypass the specialized AV junction [31] (Fig. 6.12). In these cases, the occurrence of atrial fibrillation even paroxysmal, favored by right atrial dilatation due to tricuspid valve dysfunction, may turn into ventricular fibrillation, due to a short refractory period of the working myocardium of the anomalous AVpathway.

6.4   Image Gallery

Fig. 6.1 Arrhythmic sudden cardiac death due to aortic valve stenosis in a 9-year-old girl during gymnastic activity. View of the aortic root shows bicuspid aortic valve stenosed by thickened and dysplastic cusps

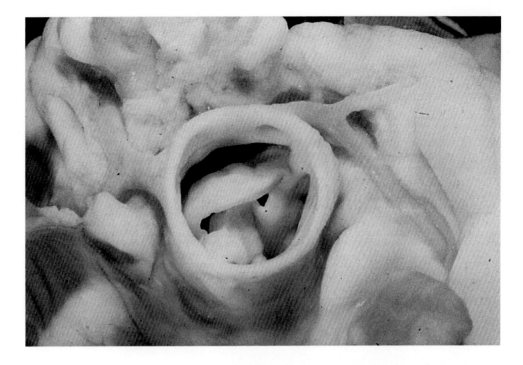

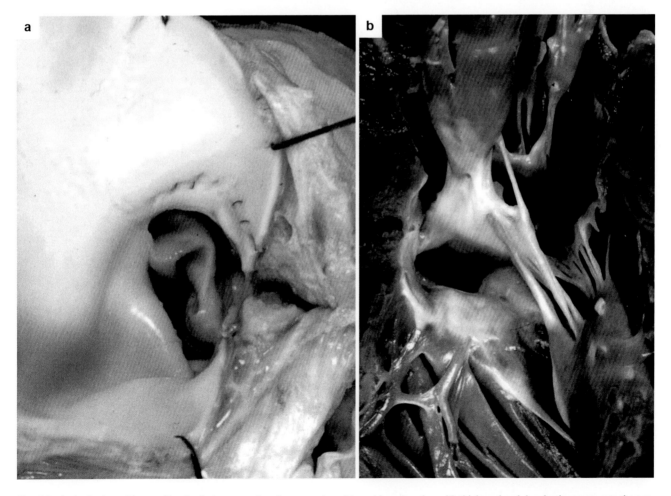

Fig. 6.2 Arrhythmic sudden cardiac death due to aortic valve stenosis in a 17-year-old boy who had a surgical commissurotomy of the aortic valve when he was a child. (**a**) View of the aortic root shows a stenotic bicuspid aortic valve with thickened and dysplastic cusps: note the previous aortotomy. (**a**, **b**) View of the left ventricular outflow tract from below with endocardial subaortic septal plaque

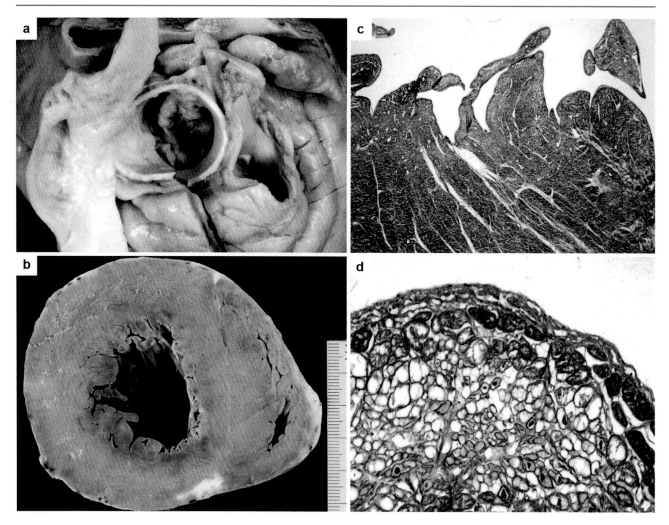

Fig. 6.3 Arrhythmic sudden cardiac death due to aortic valve stenosis in a 25-year-old drug addict male (**a**) View of the aortic root shows a stenotic, grossly malformed bicuspid aortic valve with calcified vegetations due to previous endocarditis. (**b**) Transverse section of the heart shows a concentric left ventricular hypertrophy with subendocardial ischemic damage. (**c**) The histology of the left ventricular myocardium discloses subendocardial scarring (Heidenhain trichrome). (**d**) At higher magnification, ischemic myocytolysis is visible (Heidenhain trichrome)

Fig. 6.4 Mechanical sudden cardiac death due to aortic dissection and cardiac tamponade in a 17-year-old boy with bicuspid aortic valve and isthmic coarctation. (**a**) Large intimal tear in the ascending aorta, a couple of centimeters above a bicuspid aortic valve. (**b**) Coarctation of the aortic isthmus. (**c**) Histology shows disruption of the elastic lamellae in the tunica media (Weigert–van Gieson)

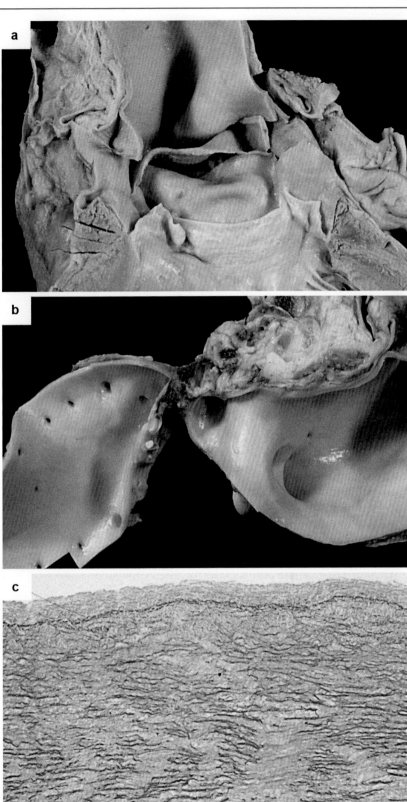

Fig. 6.5 Mechanical sudden cardiac death due to aortic dissection and cardiac tamponade in a 24-year-old man with bicuspid aortic valve. (**a**) Spontaneous intimal laceration and dissection of the ascending aorta in a heart with a normally functioning bicuspid aortic valve. (**b**) Massive fragmentation and loss of elastic lamellae of the aortic tunica media (Weigert–van Gieson)

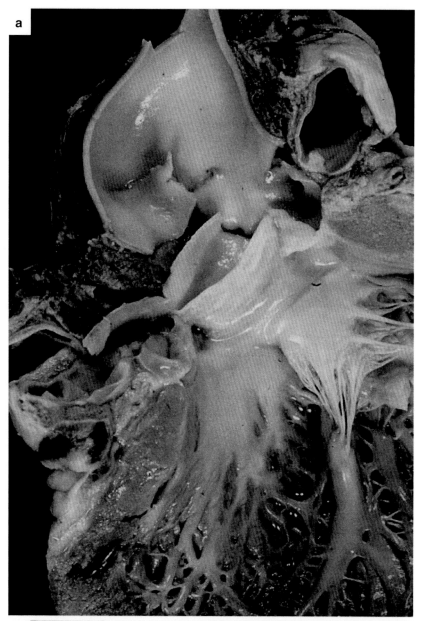

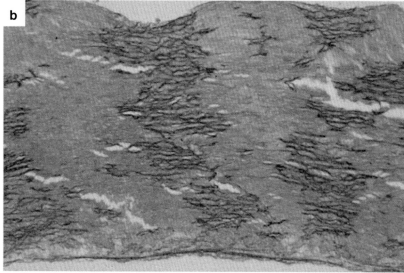

Fig. 6.6 Mechanical sudden cardiac death due to aortic dissection and cardiac tamponade in a 36-year-old man with bicuspid aortic valve. (**a**) Spontaneous intimal laceration 1 cm above the aortic valve commissures: note the bicuspid aortic valve with a raphe and the dissection of a dilated ascending aorta. (**b**) Dissection of the aortic tunica media at histology (Weigert–van Gieson)

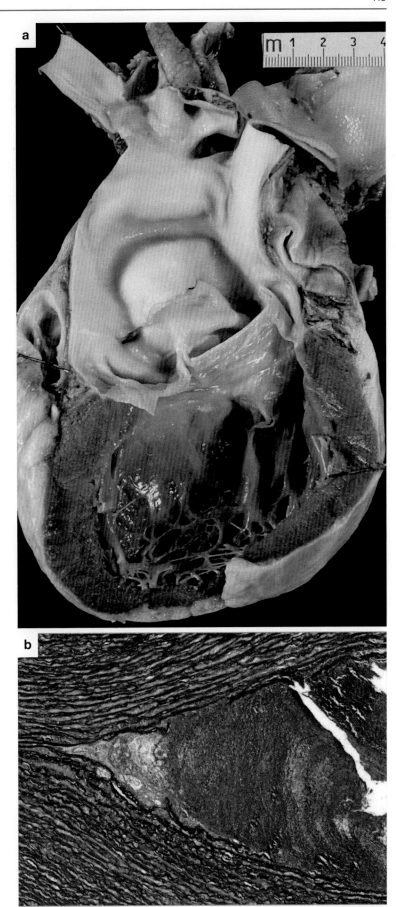

Fig. 6.7 Mechanical sudden cardiac death due to aortic dissection and cardiac tamponade in a 28-year-old boy with Marfan syndrome. (**a**) Note the oblique intimal tear in the ascending aorta just 1 cm above the commissures of the aortic valve cusps. (**b**) Histology shows severe mucoid extracellular matrix accumulation in the tunica media (Alcian PAS)

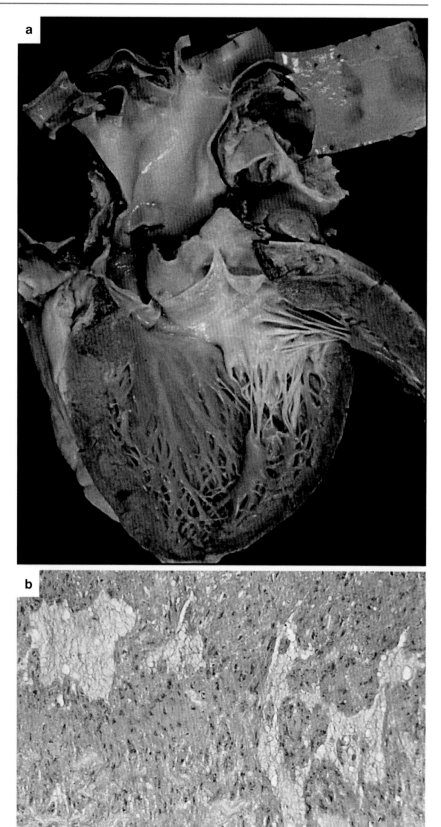

Fig. 6.8 Mechanical sudden cardiac death due to aortic dissection and cardiac tamponade in a 31-year-old boy with Marfan syndrome. (**a**) Hugely enlarged ascending aorta with disappearance of the sino-tubular junction: note the large intimal tear in the ascending aorta, a couple of centimeters above the aortic valve commissures. (**b**) Histology shows severe loss and disruption of the elastic lamellae in the tunica media (Weigert–van Gieson)

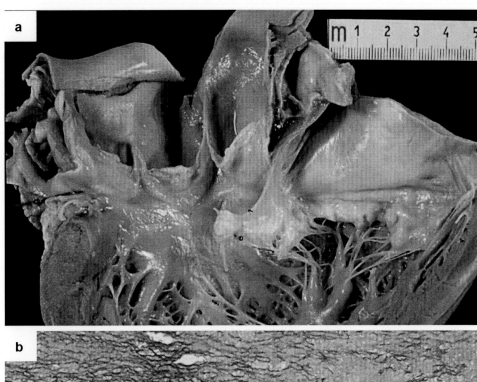

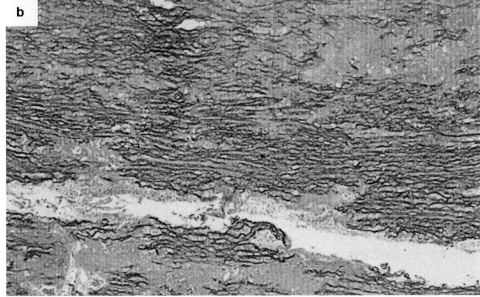

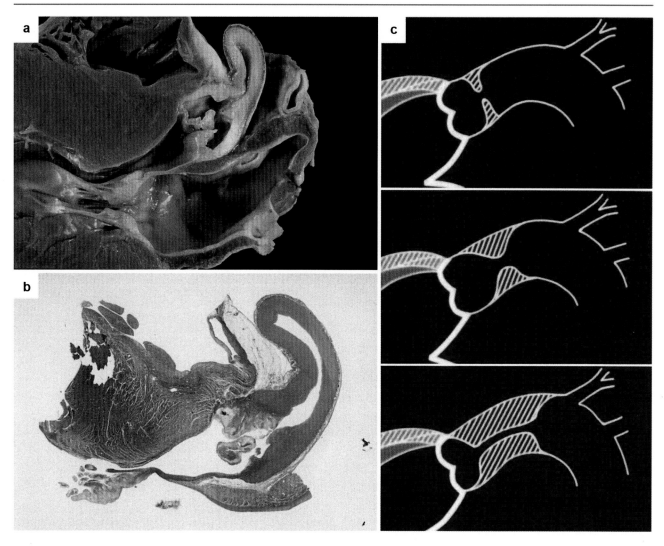

Fig. 6.9 Arrhythmic sudden cardiac death due to supravalvular aortic stenosis in a 5-year-old child on effort. (**a**) Parasternal long-axis cut of the heart: note the narrowing of the ascending aorta due to thickened aortic wall. (**b**) Corresponding panoramic histology, with thickened and dysplastic elastic tunica media and secondary aortic valve cups thickening (Weigert–van Gieson). (**c**) Diagram of the three types of supravalvular aortic stenosis: discrete membranous, hourglass, and tubular due to a diffuse, elongated narrowing

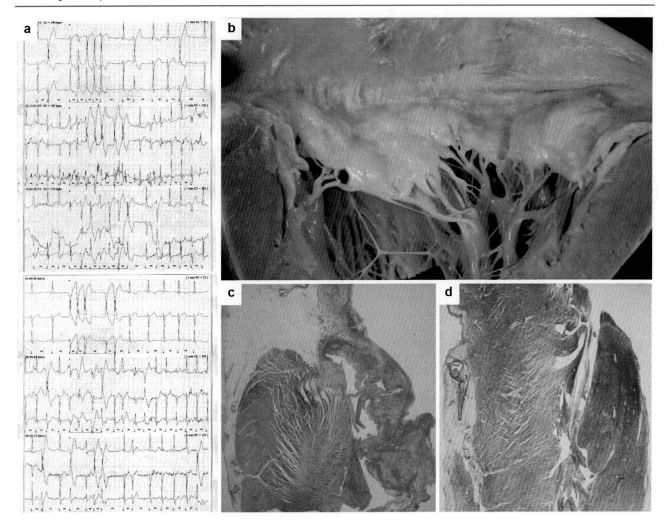

Fig. 6.10 Arrhythmic sudden cardiac death due to mitral valve prolapse in a 36-year-old woman with in vivo diagnosis. (**a**) At 24 h Holter-ECG non-sustained ventricular tachycardia. (**b**) At gross examination, myxomatous degeneration of both leaflets of the mitral valve, with elongated chordae and leaflet hoodings, is visible. (**c**, **d**) At histology, severe myxoid thickening of the posterior mitral valve leaflet and myocardial fibrosis of the LV infero-basal wall and papillary muscle (Heidenhain trichrome)

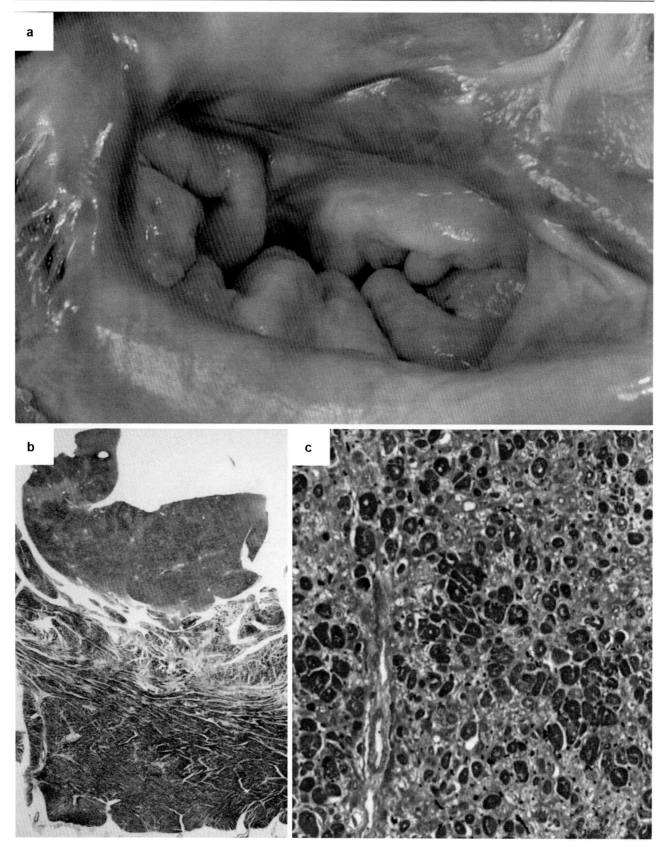

Fig. 6.11 Arrhythmic sudden cardiac death due to mitral valve prolapse in a 32-year-old man. (**a**) View of the left atrial cavity: note the mitral valve with thickened and ballooning leaflets. (**b**) Panoramic histology of the left ventricle free wall and papillary muscle shows replacement-type fibrosis (Heidenhain trichrome). (**c**) Close-up of **b** (Heidenhain trichrome)

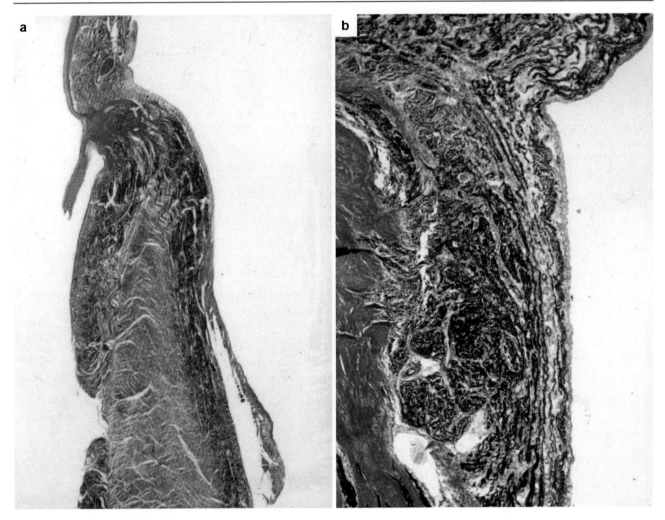

Fig. 6.12 Arrhythmic sudden cardiac death in microEbstein malformation in an 11-year-old girl who died suddenly during exercise at school. (**a**) Moderate lowering of the septal leaflet of tricuspid valve. Note that an atrial myocardial fascicle bypasses the AV node and makes contact directly with the ventricular myocardium (Heidenhain trichrome). (**b**) Another closer view shows the atrial myocardium by-passing the AV node (Heidenhain trichrome)

References

1. Basso C, Frescura C, Corrado D, Muriago M, Angelini A, Daliento L, Thiene G. Congenital heart disease and sudden death in the young. Hum Pathol. 1995;26:1065–72.
2. Thiene G, Ho SY. Aortic root pathology and sudden death in youth: review of anatomical varieties. Appl Pathol.1986;4:237-45
3. Roberts WC, Ko JM. Frequency by decades of unicuspid, bicuspid, and tricuspid aortic valves in adults having isolated aortic valve replacement for aortic stenosis, with or without associated aortic regurgitation. Circulation. 2005;111:920–5.
4. Cheitlin MD, Fenoglio JJ, McAllister HA, Davia JE, DeCastro CM. Congenital aortic stenosis secondary to dysplasia of congenital bicuspid aortic valve without commissural fusion. Am J Cardiol. 1978;42:102–7.
5. Pomerance A. Pathogenesis of aortic stenosis and its relation to age. Br Heart J. 1972;34:569.
6. Thiene G, Carturan E, Corrado D, Basso C. Prevention of sudden cardiac death in the young and in athletes: dream or reality? Cardiovasc Pathol. 2010;19:207–17.
7. Roberts CS, Roberts WC. Dissection of the aorta associated with congenital malformation of the aortic valve. J Am Coll Cardiol. 1991;17:712–6.
8. Edwards WD, Leaf DS, Edwards JE. Dissecting aortic aneurysm associated with congenital bicuspid aortic valve. Circulation. 1978;57:1022–5.
9. Nistri S, Grande-Allen J, Noale M, Basso C, Siviero P, Maggi S, Crepaldi G, Thiene G. Aortic elasticity and size in bicuspid aortic valve syndrome. Eur Heart J. 2008;15:472–9.
10. Nistri S, Porciani MC, Attanasio M, Abbate R, Gensini GF, Pepe G. Association of Marfan syndrome and bicuspid aortic valve: frequency and outcome. Int J Cardiol. 2012;15:324–5.
11. Kappetein AP, Gittenberger-de Groot AC, Zwinderman AH, Rohmer J, Poelmann RE, Huysmans HA. The neural crest as a possible pathogenetic factor in coarctation of the aorta and bicuspid aortic valve. J Thorac Cardiovasc Surg. 1991;102:830-6
12. Morrow AG, Waldhausen JA, Peters RL, Blood-Well RD, Braunwald E. Supravalvular aortic stenosis. Clinical, hemodynamic and pathologic observations. Circulation. 1959;20:1003–10.
13. Williams JCP, Barratt Boyes BG, Lowe JB. Supravalvular aortic stenosis. Circulation. 1961;24:1311–8.
14. Morris CA, Loker J, Ensing G, Stock AD. Supravalvular aortic stenosis cosegregates with a familial 6; 7 translocation which disrupts the elastin gene. Am J Med Genet. 1993;46:737–44.
15. Hayek E, Gring CN, Griffin BP. Mitral valve prolapse. Lancet. 2005;365:507–18.
16. Sriram CS, Syed FF, Ferguson ME, Johnson JN, Enriquez-Sarano M, Cetta F, Cannon BC, Asirvatham SJ, Ackerman MJ. Malignant bileaflet mitral valve prolapse syndrome in patients with otherwise idiopathic out-of-hospital cardiac arrest. J Am Coll Cardiol. 2013;62:222–30.
17. Basso C, Perazzolo Marra M, Rizzo S, De Lazzari M, Giorgi B, Cipriani A, Frigo AC, Rigato I, Migliore F, Pilichou K, Bertaglia E, Cacciavillani L, Bauce B, Corrado D, Thiene G, Iliceto S. Arrhythmic mitral valve prolapse and sudden cardiac death. Circulation. 2015;132:556–66.
18. Salazar AE, Edwards JE. Friction lesions of ventricular endocardium: relation to chordae tendineae of mitral valve. Arch Pathol. 1970;90:364–76.
19. Kligfield P, Levy D, Devereux RB, Savage DD. Arrhythmias and sudden death in mitral valve prolapse. Am Heart J. 1987;113:1316–23.
20. Bharati S, Granston AS, Liebson PR, Loeb HS, Rosen KM, Lev M. The conduction system in mitral valve prolapse syndrome with sudden death. Am Heart J. 1981;101:667–70.
21. Jeresaty RM. The syndrome associated with mid-systolic click and-or late systolic murmur. Analysis of 32 cases. Chest. 1971;59:643–7.
22. Shappell SD, Marshall CE, Brown RE, Bruce TA. Sudden death and the familial occurrence of mid-systolic click, late systolic murmur syndrome. Circulation. 1973;48:1128–34.
23. Chesler E, King RA, Edwards JE. The myxomatous mitral valve and sudden death. Circulation. 1983;67:632–9.
24. Pocock WA, Bosman CK, Chesler E, Barlow JB, Edwards JE. Sudden death in primary mitral valve prolapse. Am Heart J. 1984; 107:378–82.
25. Dollar AL, Roberts WC. Morphologic comparison of patients with mitral valve prolapse who died suddenly with patients who died from severe valvular dysfunction or other conditions. J Am Coll Cardiol. 1991;17:921–31.
26. Farb A, Tang AL, Atkinson JB, McCarthy WF, Virmani R. Comparison of cardiac findings in patients with mitral valve prolapse who die suddenly to those who have congestive heart failure from mitral regurgitation and to those with fatal noncardiac conditions. Am J Cardiol. 1992;70:234–9.
27. Watson H. Natural history of Ebstein's anomaly of tricuspid valve in childhood and adolescence: an international cooperative study of 505 cases. Br Heart J. 1974;36:417–27.
28. Lev M, Gibson S, Miller R. Ebstein's disease with Wolff-Parkinson-White syndrome. Report of a case with histopathologic study of possible conduction pathways. Am Heart J. 1955;49:724–41.
29. Smith WM, Gallagher JJ, Kerr CR, Sealy WC, Kasell JH, Benson Jr DW, Reiter MJ, Sterba R, Grant AO. The electrophysiologic basis and management of symptomatic recurrent tachycardia in patients with Ebstein's anomaly of the tricuspid valve. Am J Cardiol. 1982;49:1223–34.
30. Thiene G, Pennelli N, Rossi L. Cardiac conduction system abnormalities as a possible cause of sudden death in young athletes. Hum Pathol. 1983;14:704–9.
31. Rossi L, Thiene G. Mild Ebstein's anomaly associated with supraventricular tachycardia and sudden death: clinicomorphologic features in 3 patients. Am J Cardiol. 1984;53:332–4.

Conduction System Disease

7.1 Preexcitation Syndromes

In the normal heart, the electrical impulse arises from the sinus node, and it is transmitted from the atria to the ventricles only through the Tawarian AV conduction axis (i.e., AV node, His bundle, and bundle branches) and Purkinje fibers, after a slowdown at the AV node, which allows the atria to empty during ventricular diastole. The AV node is located at the AV septal junction, in front of the coronary sinus and underneath the membranous septum. It consists of specialized myocardium with low speed of electrical transmission and long refractory period [1–4].

There are diseases in which the AV conduction may occur also outside the specialized axis, thus bypassing the AV node.

In Wolff–Parkinson–White syndrome, characterized by short PR interval with delta wave at the basal ECG and episodes of supraventricular tachycardia [5], there is one or more accessory pathways (also known as "Kent fascicle"), which connect directly the atrial to the ventricular myocardium, outside the specialized AV axis (Figs. 7.1 and 7.2) [6–8]. The accessory pathways consist of working myocardium, which does not delay the impulse transmission from the atria to the ventricles, because it does not possess the decremental properties typical of the specialized myocardium. Thus, the electrical impulse transmission, through the accessory pathway, may anticipate the depolarization of part of the ventricular myocardium (delta wave). It also may allow the reentry of the electrical ventricular depolarization wave to the atria, triggering a circuit of supraventricular tachycardia. If the period of refractoriness of these accessory pathways is short, the risk is that a lone atrial fibrillation may transmit the electrical impulse very fast to the ventricles (up to 1 to 1) through the anomalous bundle, thus converting into ventricular fibrillation. This is why patients affected by Wolff–Parkinson–White syndrome are at risk of SCD [9–13].

The anomalous bundle connecting the atrial to ventricular musculature is located at both the right and left AV rings, particularly in correspondence of the posterior "mural" mitral leaflet [6–8].

The bundle is thin (100–150 μ in thickness) and located close to the fibrous ring, not so far from the ventricular cavity, as to be easily ablated from the endocardial side (Fig. 7.3). Serial histological section investigation of the lateral AV ring or AV septum is needed to detect this congenital anomaly [14], which is considered the smallest structural heart defect at risk of SCD [8].

In Lown–Ganong–Levine syndrome, ventricular preexcitation occurs along the regular AV conduction axis and is characterized by a short PR interval in the absence of delta wave [15]. The AV conduction is accelerated ("enhanced AV conduction") because of a congenitally hypoplastic AV node [16] or of the existence of an anomalous pathway by passing the AV node (site of slow down) and connecting directly to the His bundle (Figs. 7.4 and 7.5) [2–4]. These atrio-hissian anomalous pathways (James or Brechenmacher's fascicles) consist also of working myocardium, which has high-speed properties for impulse conduction and short refractory period, allowing both preexcitation and reentry tachycardia, as well as triggering ventricular fibrillation in the occurrence of atrial fibrillation [1–4].

Anyway, in the presence of ventricular preexcitation, the trigger of atrial fibrillation, degenerating into ventricular fibrillation, remains intriguing. Episodes of supraventricular tachycardia, which occasionally turns into ventricular fibrillation, have been hypothesized. Furthermore, atrial myocarditis, possibly triggering paroxysmal atrial fibrillation, has been demonstrated in young people dying suddenly (Fig. 7.6) [8]. In both conditions, the anomalous pathway of working myocardium should possess a very short refractory period to convert atrial fibrillation into ventricular fibrillation.

7.2 Atrioventricular Block

The AV block in the young, at risk of asystole and cardiac arrest, may be congenital or acquired. Among congenital blocks, the most frequent is the one observed in children of

© Springer-Verlag Milan 2016
G. Thiene et al., *Sudden Cardiac Death in the Young and Athletes: Text Atlas of Pathology and Clinical Correlates*,
DOI 10.1007/978-88-470-5776-0_7

mother with systemic lupus erythematosus [17, 18]. Both the sinus node and AV node appear destroyed by an inflammatory necrotic process, most probably immune in origin, with lymphocytic infiltrates, fibrosis, and even calcification. The other congenital non-Lupus-related AV block is the consequence of a maldevelopment of the specialized AV axis, with a lack of connection between the AV node and the His bundle. It may be observed in otherwise normal hearts or in hearts with complex congenital heart diseases, like congenitally corrected transposition and single ventricle [19–21].

The acquired AV block, which appears early in young age, presents a quite different substrate (Lenegre's disease) [22]. The histopathology consists of a fibrosis of the bifurcating bundle and proximal left and right bundle branches, whereas the surrounding working myocardium appears intact (Fig. 7.7). A cardiomyopathy of the specialized conducting tissues has been postulated [23].

Some of these cases with acquired AV block are heredofamilial, and mutations in the SCN5A gene encoding sodium ion channel have been discovered through molecular investigations (Fig. 7.8) [24]. By the way, Brugada syndrome, which is also explained by SCN5A mutations, is characterized by PR prolongation and right bundle branch block, which at histological examination appears to have an organic substrate, i.e., fibrosis of the bifurcating bundle and proximal right bundle branch [25].

7.3   Cardiac Tumors

Cardiac tumors are rare and might exceptionally cause SCD due to an either mechanical (for instance, endocavitary myxoma or rhabdomyoma with hemodynamic compromise – see Chap. 3) or arrhythmic pathophysiologic mechanism [26, 27].

As far as the latter group is concerned, we will take into consideration cystic tumor of the AV node, Purkinje cell tumor, and cardiac fibroma, which are reported as a cause of SCD in the young.

The cystic tumor of the AV node (also known as Tawarioma or celothelioma of the AV node) represents an embryonal inclusion in the heart's center of mesodermal tissue and is characterized by heterotopic epithelial replacement of the AV node with multicystic appearance. It grows more or less rapidly with tubule-cystic features as to produce congenital, juvenile, or adult complete supra-hissian AV block [26, 28] (Fig. 7.9).

The Purkinje cell tumor (also known as histiocytoid cardiomyopathy, idiopathic infantile cardiomyopathy, purkinjoma) is a rare cause of severe and intractable tachyarrhythmias early in infancy [26, 29–33]. The masses grossly appear as focal yellowish nodules or areas of discoloration, ranging in size from 1 mm to 1.5 cm in diameter, most commonly located along the conduction system and within the working myocardium of the left ventricle. Microscopically, these masses contain large oval cardiac myocytes with a coarse granular pale cytoplasm (Fig. 7.10).

Cardiac fibroma is the second most frequent type of cardiac tumor in the pediatric age. Macroscopically, the fibroma usually is a single, solid, well-defined, whitish, and whorled not encapsulated mass, almost invariably intramural, and usually located in the right or left ventricular free walls, or in the interventricular septum. At histology, the fibroma consists of a homogeneous mass of fibroblasts mixed with abundant extracellular matrix, which often entraps cardiomyocytes. These tumors may reach huge dimensions, even up to 8 cm of diameter, as to obstruct the ventricular cavity and cause hemodynamic symptoms/signs. When located in the central fibrous body, the fibroma might compress the His bundle and induce AV block [34, 35]. However, fibroma often accounts for life-threatening ventricular arrhythmias due to reentry of the intraventricular electrical impulse.

7.4   Image Gallery

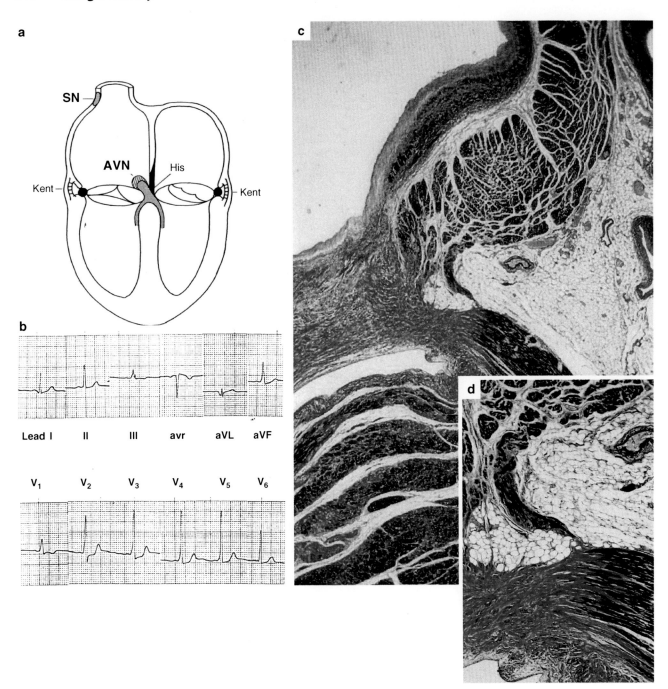

Fig. 7.1 Arrhythmic cardiac arrest in a 35-year-old man with an in vivo diagnosis of Wolff–Parkinson–White syndrome. (**a**) Diagrams illustrating the normal specialized sinus node (SN) and atrioventricular node (AVN) and junction as well as the accessory AV connections (Kent fascicles) which may be situated at the septal and lateral levels; (**b**) 12-lead ECG tracing with short PR interval and delta wave; (**c**) the Kent fascicle, located close to the endocardium, joins the working atrial and ventricular myocardium (Heidenhain trichrome); (**d**) close-up of (**c**)

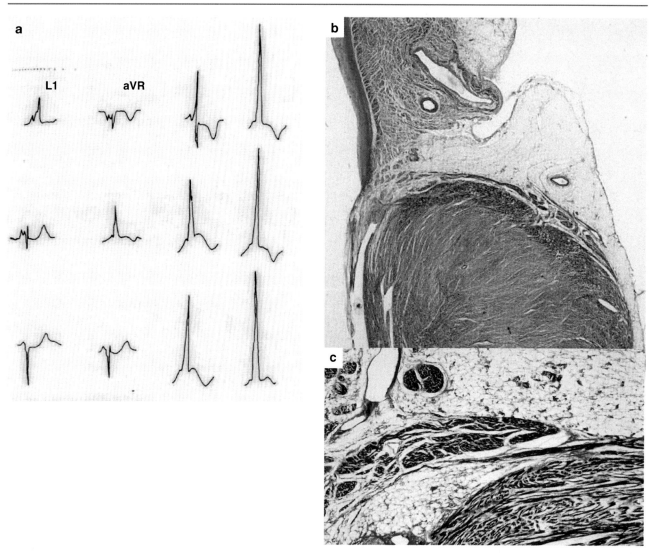

Fig. 7.2 Arrhythmic cardiac arrest in a 9-year-old boy with an in vivo diagnosis of Wolff– Parkinson–White syndrome. (**a**) 12-lead ECG tracing with short PR interval and delta wave. (**b**) A section of the left lateral AV ring shows the Kent fascicle, joining the working atrial and ventricular myocardium (Heidenhain trichrome); (**c**) close-up of (**b**)

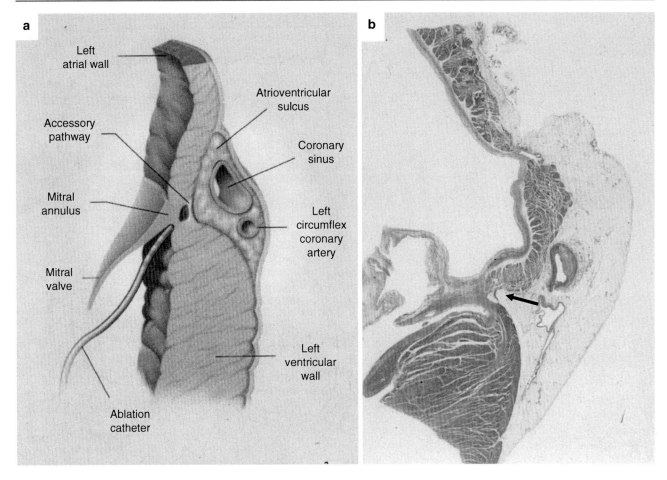

Fig. 7.3 (**a**) Diagram illustrating the left AV junction. The location of the accessory AV connection (Kent fascicle) close to the endocardium is easily reachable by the ablation catheter. (**b**) Panoramic histology note the Kent fascicle located close to the endocardium (*arrow*) (same case as Fig. 7.1) (Heidenhain trichrome)

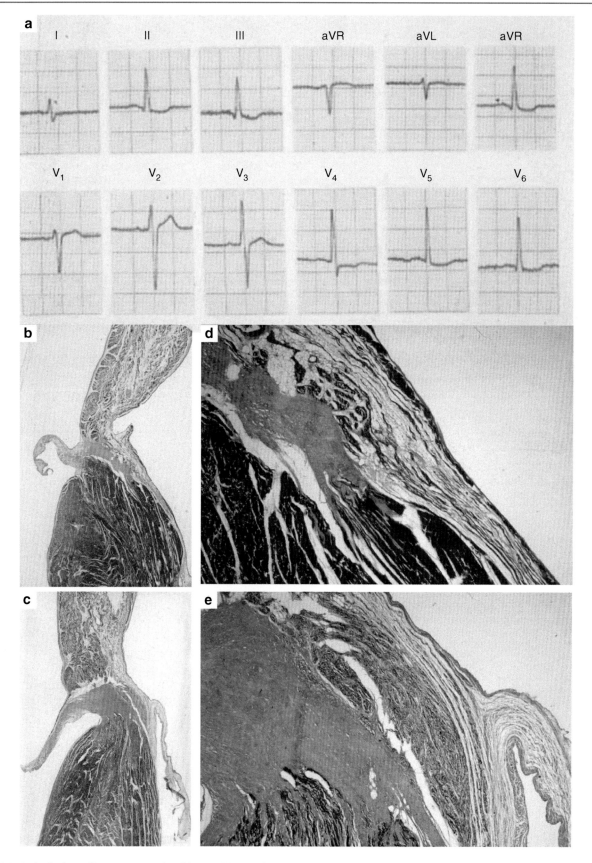

Fig. 7.4 Arrhythmic cardiac arrest at rest in a 34-year-old man with an in vivo diagnosis of Lown–Ganong–Levine syndrome. (**a**) 12-lead ECG tracing with short PR interval in the absence of delta wave. (**b**) Histological section of the septal AV junction, at the level of the AV node: note the hypoplastic AV node as compared to a normal-sized AV node in a control subject (**c**) (Heidenhain trichrome). (**d**, **e**) Close-up of (**b**) and (**c**), respectively (Heidenhain trichrome)

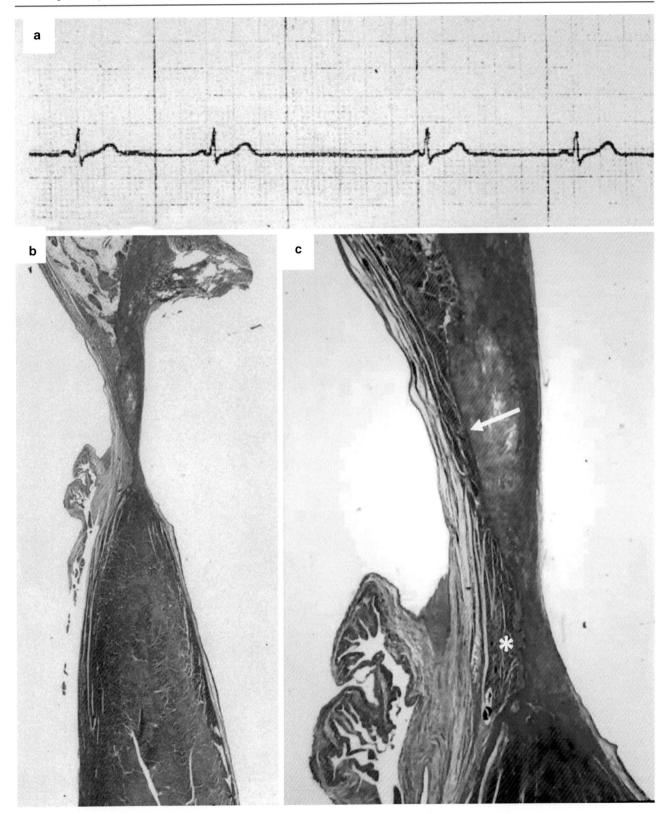

Fig. 7.5 Arrhythmic cardiac arrest while sleeping in a 21-year-old man with an in vivo diagnosis of Lown–Ganong–Levine syndrome. (**a**) ECG tracing (D1 lead) with short PR interval in the absence of delta wave. (**b**) Section of the septal AV junction, at the level of the AV conducting tissue: note the anomalous pathway (James fascicle, *arrow*) by-passing the AV node and connecting directly to the His bundle (*) (Heidenhain trichrome). (**c**) Close-up of (**b**) (Heidenhain trichrome)

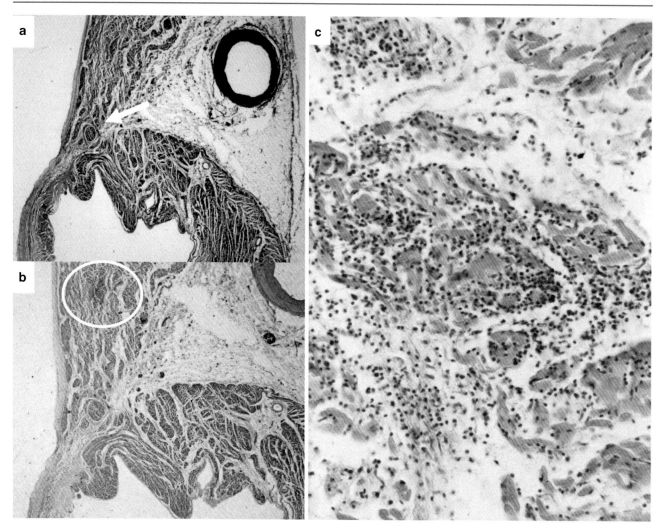

Fig. 7.6 Arrhythmic cardiac arrest in a 19-year-old man with an in vivo diagnosis of Wolff– Parkinson–White syndrome and atrial myocarditis. (**a**) Serial section of the left AV ring shows the accessory connection (*arrow*) (Kent fascicle). (**b**) Same as figure (**a**): note the inflammatory cells infiltrate in the atrial myocardium (*circled area*), close to the anomalous pathway (hematoxylin–eosin). (**c**) Close-up of inflammatory infiltrate of the atrial myocardium (hematoxylin–eosin)

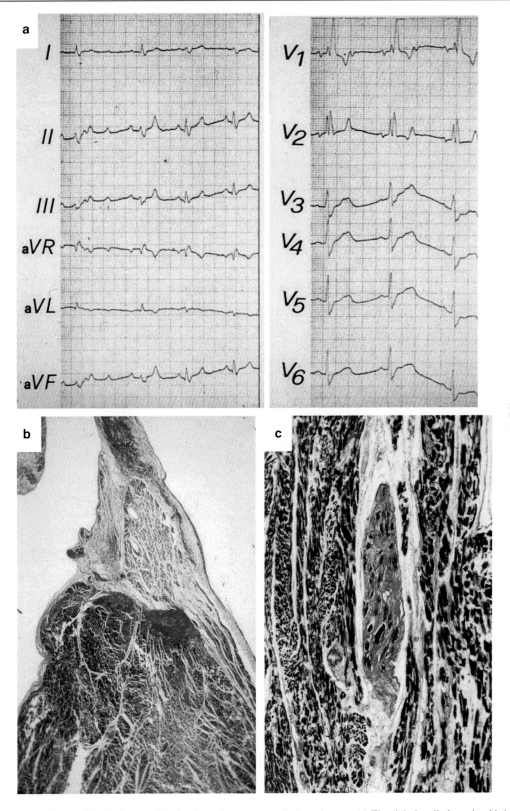

Fig. 7.7 Arrhythmic sudden cardiac death caused by Lenègre disease with AV block in a 55-year-old man. (**a**) An ECG shows complete AV block in peripheral leads and second-degree AV block in precordial leads. (**b**) Sclero-atrophy of the branching bundle at the origin of the left bundle branch stem. (**c**) The right bundle branch with intramyocardial course shows almost complete replacement by fibrous tissue (**b** and **c**, Heidenhain trichrome)

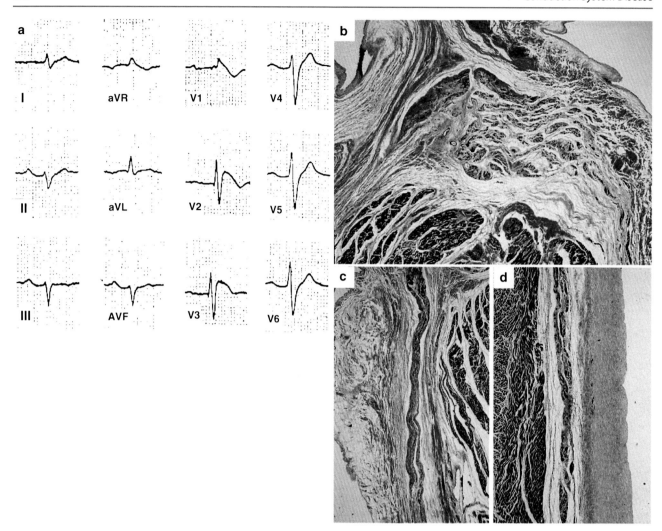

Fig. 7.8 Arrhythmic sudden cardiac death in a 40-year-old man, with Brugada sydrome ECG, recurrent syncope and previous cardiac arrest. (**a**) 12-lead ECG shows sinus rhythm, first-degree AV block (PR interval 220 ms), right bundle branch block with left-axis deviation, coved-type ST segment elevation, and inverted T waves in the right precordial leads. (**b**) On serial histological sections of the specialized conduction system, severe fibrosis of the bifurcating His bundle and sclerotic interruption of right and left bundle branches are visible in keeping with Lenègre disease (**c, d**) (**b, c, d**, Heidenhain trichrome)

Fig. 7.9 Cystic tumor of the AV node (tawarioma): note the multi-cystic neoplasm at the level of the AV node (Heidenhain trichrome)

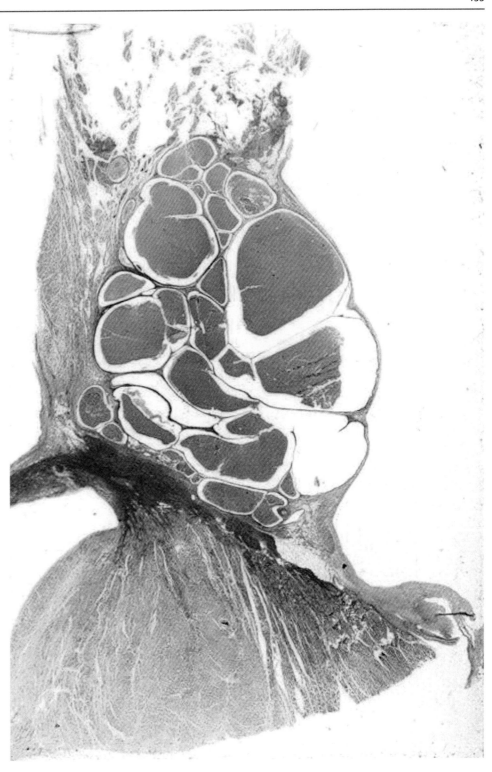

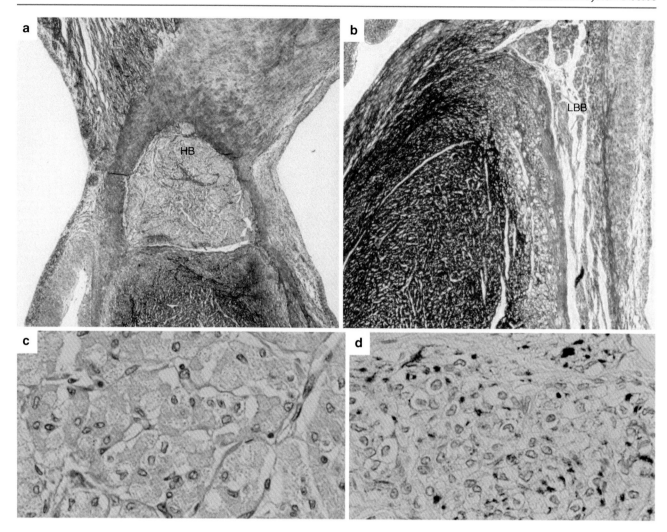

Fig. 7.10 Purkinje cell tumor in a 1-month-old child with junctional ectopic tachycardia. (**a**) Histology of the His bundle (HB) with large, vacuolated Purkinje-like cells (Heidenhain trichrome). (**b**) Purkinje-like cells are also visible within the working myocardium of the ventricular septum (*asterisc*), close to the left bundle branch (LBB) (Heidenhain trichrome). (**c**) At higher magnification, the cells appear swollen and pale, with vacuolated, finely granular cytoplasm (hematoxylin–eosin). (**d**) At immunohistochemistry, the cells are positive for myocardial markers (desmin).

References

1. Basso C, Ho Y, Rizzo S, Thiene G. Anatomic and histopathologic characteristics of the conductive tissues of the heart, chapter 4. In: Gussak I, Antzelevitch C, editors. Electrical diseases of the heart. London: Springer; 2013. p. 47–71.
2. Rossi L. Neuroanatomopathology of the cardiovascular system. In: Kulbertus H, Franck G, editors. Neurocardiology. NY, Futura: Mount Kisko; 1988. p. 25.
3. Rossi L. Histopathology of cardiac arrhythmias. Philadelphia: Lea & Febiger; 1979.
4. Davies MJ. Pathology of conducting tissue of the heart. London: Butterworths; 1971.
5. Wolff L, Parkinson J, White PD. Bundle-branch block with short P-R interval in healthy young people prone to paroxysmal tachycardia. Am Heart J. 1930;5:685–704.
6. Anderson RH, Becker AE, Brechenmacher C, Davies MJ, Rossi L. Ventricular preexcitation. A proposed nomenclature for its substrates. Eur J Cardiol. 1975;3:27–36.
7. Becker AE, Anderson RH, Durrer D, Wellens HJ. The anatomical substrates of Wolff-Parkinson-White syndrome. A clinicopathologic correlation in seven patients. Circulation. 1978;57:870–9.
8. Basso C, Corrado D, Rossi L, Thiene G. Ventricular preexcitation in children and young adults: atrial myocarditis as a possible trigger of sudden death. Circulation. 2001;103:269–75.
9. Klein GJ, Prystowsky EN, Yee R, Sharma AD, Laupacis A. Asymptomatic Wolff-Parkinson-White: should we intervene? Circulation. 1989;80:1902–5.
10. Leitch JW, Klein GJ, Yee R, Murdock C. Prognostic value of electrophysiologic testing in asymptomatic patients with Wolff-Parkinson-White pattern. Circulation. 1990;82:1718–23.
11. Klein GJ, Bashore TM, Sellers TD, Pritchett EL, Smith WM, Gallagher JJ. Ventricular fibrillation in the Wolff-Parkinson-White syndrome. N Engl J Med. 1979;301:1080–5.
12. Wellens HJJ, Durrer D. Wolff-Parkinson-White syndrome and atrial fibrillation. Relation between refractory period of accessory pathway and ventricular rate during atrial fibrillation. Am J Cardiol. 1974;34:777–82.
13. Wellens HJJ, Bar FW, Farre J. Sudden death in the Wolff-Parkinson-White syndrome. In: Kulbertus H, Wellens HJJ, editors. Sudden death. Boston: Martinus Nijhoff; 1980. p. 392.
14. Basso C, Burke M, Fornes P, Gallagher PJ, de Gouveia RH, Sheppard M, Thiene G, van der Wal A, Association for European Cardiovascular Pathology. Guidelines for autopsy investigation of sudden cardiac death. Virchows Arch. 2008;452:11–8.
15. Lown B, Ganong WF, Levine SA. The syndrome of short P-R interval, normal QRS complex and paroxysmal rapid heart action. Circulation. 1952;5:693–706.
16. Ometto R, Thiene G, Corrado D, Vincenzi M, Rossi L. Enhanced A-V nodal conduction (Lown-Ganong-Levine syndrome) by congenitally hypoplastic A-V node. Eur Heart J. 1992;13:1579–84.
17. Chameides L, Truex RC, Vetter V, Rashkind WJ, Galioto Jr FM, Noonan JA. Association of maternal systemic lupus erythematosus with congenital complete heart block. N Engl J Med. 1977;297:1204–7.
18. Angelini A, Moreolo GS, Ruffatti A, Milanesi O, Thiene G. Calcification of the atrioventricular node in a fetus affected by congenital complete heart block. Circulation. 2002;105:1254–5.
19. Daliento L, Corrado D, Buja G, John N, Nava A, Thiene G. Rhythm and conduction disturbances in isolated, congenitally corrected transposition of the great arteries. Am J Cardiol. 1986;58:314–8.
20. Thiene G, Nava A, Rossi L. The conduction system in corrected transposition with situs inversus. Eur J Cardiol. 1977;6:57–70.
21. Rossi L, Montella S, Frescura C, Thiene G. Congenital atrioventricular block in right atrial isomerism (asplenia). A case due to atrionodal discontinuity. Chest. 1984;85:578–80.
22. Lenegre J. Etiology and pathology of bilateral bundle branch block in relation to complete heart block. Prog Cardiovasc Dis. 1964;6:409–44.
23. Corrado D, Nava A, Buja G, Martini B, Fasoli G, Oselladore L, Turrini P, Thiene G. Familial cardiomyopathy underlies syndrome of right bundle branch block, ST segment elevation and sudden death. J Am Coll Cardiol. 1996;27:443–8.
24. Schott JJ, Alshinawi C, Kyndt F, Probst V, Hoorntje TM, Hulsbeek M, Wilde AA, Escande D, Mannens MM, Le Marec H. Cardiac conduction defects associate with mutations in SCN5A. Nat Genet. 1999;23:20–1.
25. Kyndt F, Probst V, Potet F, Demolombe S, Chevallier JC, Baro I, Moisan JP, Boisseau P, Schott JJ, Escande D, Le Marec H. Novel SCN5A mutation leading either to isolated cardiac conduction defect or Brugada syndrome in a large French family. Circulation. 2001;104:3081–6.
26. Basso C, Valente M, Thiene G. Cardiac tumor pathology. New York: Humana Press; 2013.
27. Cina SJ, Smialek JE, Burke AP, Virmani R, Hutchins GM. Primary cardiac tumors causing sudden death: a review of the literature. Am J Forensic Med Pathol. 1996;17:271–81.
28. James TN, Galakhov I, De subitaneis mortibus. XXVI. Fatal electrical instability of the heart associated with benign congenital polycystic tumor of the atrioventricular node. Circulation. 1977;56:667–78.
29. Rossi L, Piffer R, Turolla E, Frigerio B, Coumel P, James TN. Multifocal Purkinje tumor of the heart. Occurrence with other anatomic abnormalities in the atrioventricular junction of an infant with junctional tachycardia, Lown-Ganong-Levine Syndrome and sudden death. Chest. 1985;87:340–5.
30. Rizzo S, Basso C, Buja G, Valente M, Thiene G. Multifocal Purkinje-like hamartoma and junctional ectopic tachycardia with a rapidly fatal outcome in a newborn. Heart Rhythm. 2014;11:1264–6.
31. James TN, Beeson 2nd CW, Sherman EB, Mowry RW, Clinical conference: De subitaneis mortibus. XIII. Multifocal Purkinje cell tumors of the heart. Circulation. 1975;52:333–44.
32. Malhotra V, Ferrans VJ, Virmani R. Infantile histiocytoid cardiomyopathy: three cases and literature review. Am Heart J. 1994;128:1009–21.
33. Ottaviani G, Matturri L, Rossi L, Lavezzi AM, James TN. Multifocal cardiac Purkinje cell tumor in infancy. Europace. 2004;6:138–41.
34. James TN, Carlson DJL, Marshall TK, De subitaneis mortibus. I. Fibroma compressing His bundle. Circulation. 1973;48:428–33.
35. James TN. Chance and sudden death. J Am Coll Cardiol. 1983;1:164–83.

Congenital Heart Disease

The natural history of some congenital heart diseases can be featured by electrical instability at risk of SCD, both at rest and on effort.

By definition, congenital heart disease is a structural defect present at birth. As such, genetically determined cardiomyopathies, like hypertrophic and arrhythmogenic, in which the phenotypic expression occurs in childhood, should not strictly be regarded as congenital heart diseases. They have been treated and illustrated separately under the chapter of cardiomyopathies.

The most life-threatening congenital heart diseases, at risk of SCD, are hidden and poorly symptomatic structural defects, quite difficult to detect at physical examination. This is the case of bicuspid aortic valve, congenital coronary artery anomalies with origin still from the aorta, but in the wrong sinus, and ventricular preexcitation due to AV accessory pathways (Wolff–Parkinson–White syndrome) [1]. These congenital malformations have been already discussed and illustrated within the chapters of valve, coronary, and conduction system disease, respectively.

Among overt congenital heart diseases, those with septal defects complicated by pulmonary vascular disease (Eisenmenger syndrome) have been reported in SCD series. SCD is indeed one of the modes of death in these patients (Figs. 8.1 and 8.2) [2].

The most electrically vulnerable hearts of subjects affected by congenital malformations are those which had undergone surgical repair. Injury of the AV conduction system during operation and/or myocardial scars following ventriculotomy or implantation of a conduit to reconstruct the continuity between the right ventricle and the pulmonary artery, like in tetralogy of Fallot, double-outlet right ventricle, truncus arteriosus, and transposition with pulmonary stenosis, are the usual arrhythmogenic substrates [1].

In complete transposition of the great arteries, atrial switch operation may also jeopardize the electrical cardiac stability with resection of the atrial septum [3]. Arterial switch repair, with reimplantation of the coronary arteries, has also sequelae in the long-term follow-up, when complicated by coronary artery stenosis at risk of ischemia and cardiac arrest [4, 5].

However, tetralogy of Fallot is the most frequently operated congenital heart disease at risk of SCD (Fig. 8.3). The arrhythmogenic substrate is a combination of right ventricular outflow tract fibrosis, because of infundibulectomy due to the closure of the ventricular septal defect and removal of subpulmonary stenosis, and of the implantation of a transannular patch for pulmonary outflow enlargement or pulmonary conduit [6–10]. Postoperative pulmonary valve incompetence may account for the right ventricular dilatation, which also contributes, together with the right ventricular myocardial fibrosis, to impair the electrical impulse transmission within the right ventricle and trigger reentrant life-threatening arrhythmias.

Finally, corrected transposition, in which the AV conduction system is congenitally displaced anteriorly along with the pulmonary outflow tract, is at risk of SCD because of congenital or acquired AV block (Figs. 8.4 and 8.5) [11, 12].

The increasing number of adult patients with congenital heart diseases (grown-up congenital heart disease-GUCH population), either successfully operated on or not, raises the need to control their cardiac electrical vulnerability [13–19]. Surgeons nowadays are fully aware of the need to avoid damaging the conduction system as well as limiting ventriculotomy only when strictly necessary. Both isolated ventricular septal defects and tetralogy of Fallot are nowadays repaired through an atrial approach, to avoid the risk of ventricular myocardial scarring.

© Springer-Verlag Milan 2016
G. Thiene et al., *Sudden Cardiac Death in the Young and Athletes: Text Atlas of Pathology and Clinical Correlates*,
DOI 10.1007/978-88-470-5776-0_8

8.1   Image Gallery

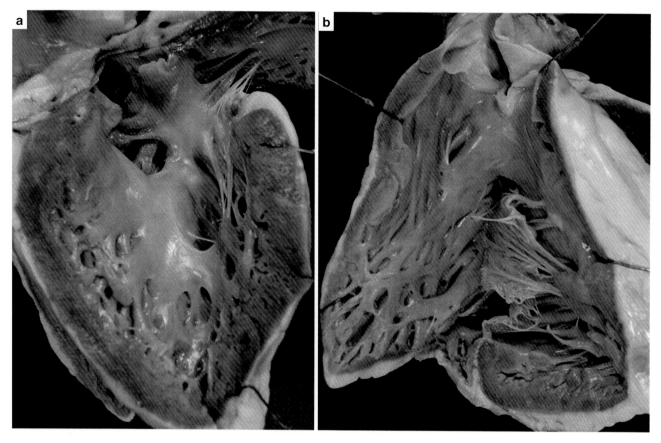

Fig. 8.1 Arrhythmic sudden cardiac death in 18-year-old boy with Eisenmenger complex. (**a**) Gross view of the perimembranous ventricular septal defect seen from the left side. The aorta is overriding the ven- tricular septum. (**b**) View of the right ventricular outflow tract with partial origin of the aorta from the right ventricle

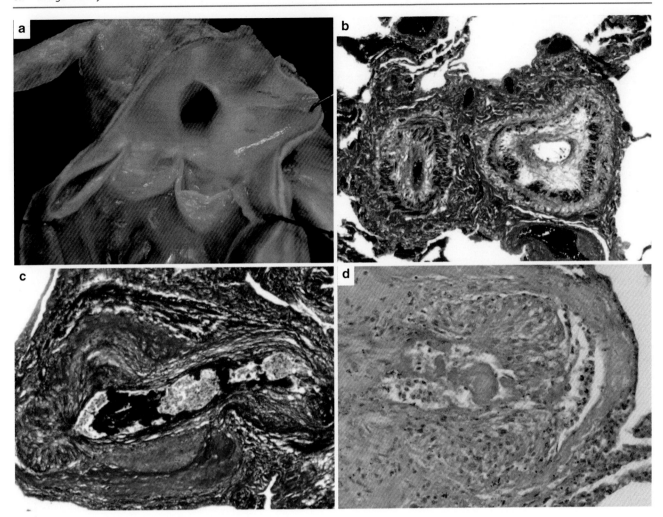

Fig. 8.2 Same case as Fig. 8.1. (**a**) Gross view of the pulmonary artery with atherosclerotic plaques in keeping with pulmonary hypertension. (**b**) Histology of the lung: small pulmonary arteries with obstructive intimal proliferation (Heidenhain trichrome). (**c**) Plexiform lesion with aneurysms of a small pulmonary artery (Heidenhain trichrome). (**d**) Glomoid proliferation and fibrinoid necrosis (hematoxylin–eosin)

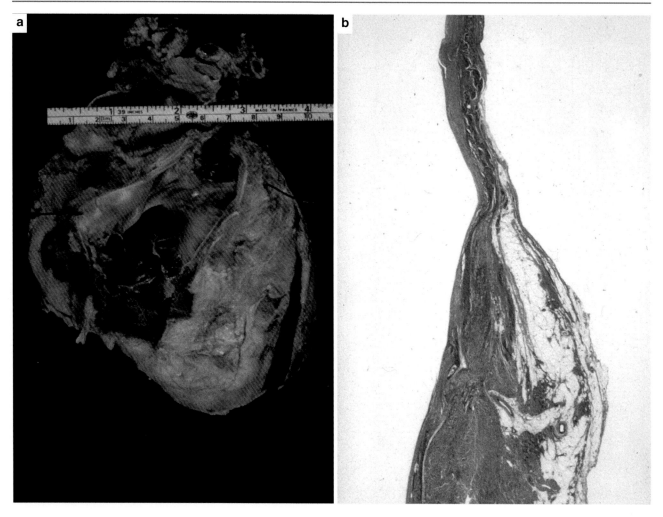

Fig. 8.3 Arrhythmic sudden cardiac death during gymnastics in a 12-year-old girl with previous surgical repair of tetralogy of Fallot. (**a**) Gross view of the right ventricular outflow tract with transannular patch and endocardial thickening. (**b**) Extensive fibrosis at histology of the pulmonary infundibulum (Heidenhain trichrome)

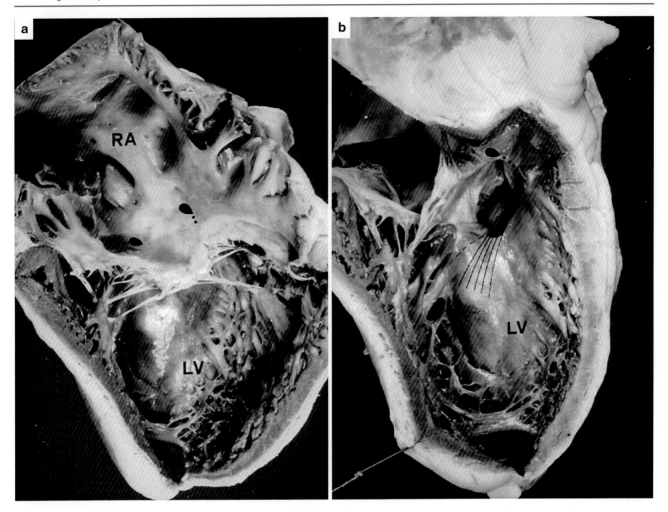

Fig. 8.4 Arrhythmic sudden cardiac death in a 54-year-old woman with corrected transposition of the great arteries. (**a**) View of the right cardiac chamber: note the AV discordance (right atrium-RA-connected to the left ventricle-LV-through the mitral valve). There are two AV nodes, but only the anterior one is connected to the ventricles. (**b**) View of the pulmonary outflow from the left ventricle-LV-: the AV node is located in the mitro-pulmonary continuity and the His bundle along the pulmonary outflow

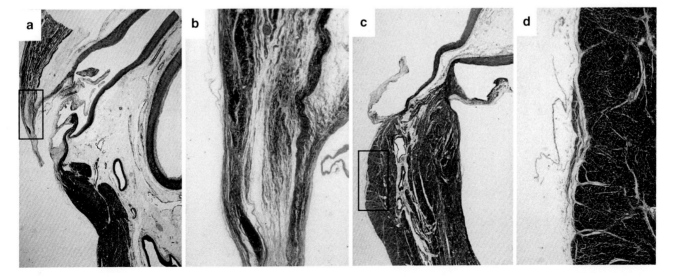

Fig. 8.5 Same case as Fig. 8.4. Histology of the AV conduction system. (**a**) The AV node (*boxed area*) is located anteriorly in the right atrium, just in front of the pulmonary outflow. (**b**) Close-up of the AV node which appears fibrotic. (**c**) The course of the His bundle (*boxed area*) is in the subendocardium on the right side of the ventricular septum, just underneath a pulmonary cusp. (**d**) Close-up of (**c**): the His bundle appears severely fibrotic, thus accounting for acquired AV block and cardiac arrest due to asystole (all Heidenhain trichrome)

References

1. Basso C, Frescura C, Corrado D, Muriago M, Angelini A, Daliento L, Thiene G. Congenital heart disease and sudden death in the young. Hum Pathol. 1995;26:1065–72.

2. Krexi D, Sheppard MN. Pulmonary hypertensive vascular changes in lungs of patients with sudden unexpected death. Emphasis on congenital heart disease, Eisenmenger syndrome, postoperative deaths and death during pregnancy and postpartum. J Clin Pathol. 2015;68:18–21.

3. Gillette PC, Kugler JD, Garson A, Gutgesell HP, Duff DF, McNamara DG. Mechanism of cardiac arrhythmias after the Mustard operation for transposition of the great arteries. Am J Cardiol. 1980;45:1225–30.

4. Murphy Jr DJ. Transposition of the great arteries: long-term outcome and current management. Curr Cardiol Rep. 2005;7:299–304.

5. Stoica S, Carpenter E, Campbell D, Mitchell M, da Cruz E, Ivy D, Lacour-Gayet F. Morbidity of the arterial switch operation. Ann Thorac Surg. 2012;93:1977–83.

6. Dunningan A, Pritzker MR, Benditt DG, Benson Jr DW. Life threatening ventricular tachycardia in late survivors of surgically corrected tetralogy of Fallot. Am J Cardiol. 1980;46:635–42.

7. Deanfield JE, Ho SY, Anderson RH, McKenna WJ, Allwork SP, Hallidie-Smith KA. Late sudden death after repair of tetralogy of Fallot: a clinicopathologic study. Circulation. 1983;67:626–31.

8. Murphy JG, Gersh BJ, Mair DD, Fuster V, McGoon MD, Ilstrup DM, McGoon DC, Kirklin JW, Danielson GK. Long-term outcome in patients undergoing surgical repair of tetralogy of Fallot. N Engl J Med. 1993;329:593–9.

9. Gatzoulis MA, Balaji S, Webber SA, Siu SC, Hokanson JS, Poile C, Rosenthal M, Nakazawa M, Moller JH, Gillette PC, Webb GD. Redington AN Risk factors for arrhythmia and sudden cardiac death late after repair of tetralogy of Fallot: a multicentre study. Lancet. 2000;356:975–81.

10. Le Gloan L, Khairy P. Management of arrhythmias in patients with tetralogy of Fallot. Curr Opin Cardiol. 2011;26:60–5.

11. Daliento L, Buja G, Corrado D, Thiene G. Complete atrioventricular block and sudden death in isolated corrected transposition. G Ital Cardiol. 1986;16:702–6.

12. Daliento L, Corrado D, Buja G, John N, Nava A, Thiene G. Rhythm and conduction disturbances in isolated, congenitally corrected transposition of the great arteries. Am J Cardiol. 1986;58:314–8.

13. Stelling JA, Danford DA, Kugler JD, Windle JR, Cheatham JP, Gumbiner CH, Latson LA, Hofschire PJ. Late potentials and inducible ventricular tachycardia in surgically repaired congenital heart disease. Circulation. 1990;82:1690–6.

14. Silka MJ, Hardy BG, Menashe VD, Morris CD. A population-based prospective evaluation of risk of sudden cardiac death after operation for common congenital heart defects. J Am Coll Cardiol. 1998;32:245–51.

15. Thiene G, Wenink AG, Frescura C, Wilkinson JL, Gallucci V, Ho SY, Mazzucco A, Anderson RH. Surgical anatomy and pathology of the conduction tissue in atrioventricular defects. J Thorac Cardiovasc Surg. 1981;82:928–37.

16. Titus JL, Daugherty GW, Edwards JE. Anatomy of the atrioventricular conduction system in ventricular septal defect. Circulation. 1963;28:72–81.

17. Okoroma EO, Guller B, Maloney JD, Weidman WH. Etiology of right bundle branch block pattern after surgical repair of ventricular septal defects. Am Heart J. 1975;90:14–8.

18. Anderson RH, Ho SY. The morphologic substrates for pediatric arrhythmias. Cardiol Young. 1991;1:159.

19. Koyak Z, Harris L, de Groot JR, Silversides CK, Oechslin EN, Bouma BJ, Budts W, Zwinderman AH, Van Gelder IC, Mulder BJ. Sudden cardiac death in adult congenital heart disease. Circulation. 2012;126:1944–54.

Ion Channel Disease

In nearly 15–20 % of SCDs in the young, a gross and histological examination of the heart fails to reveal a convincing pathological substrate which may explain the fatal outcome [1–4]. A thorough and complete autopsy, including the brain, results to be negative for an extracardiac or mechanical cardiac cause of death [5]. The heart is structurally normal and, by exclusion, the death is nothing but arrhythmic in origin. This death is known as "mors sine materia" and is frequently of familial occurrence, suggesting a hereditary genetically determined disorder [4]. Only the employment of molecular investigation may help to detect the genetic abnormality in the nucleotide DNA sequence, thus allowing to find that many SCDs sine materia are indeed ion channel diseases, now listed among nonstructural cardiomyopathies [6, 7]. Circumstances of death and the availability of the 12-lead ECG recorded during life are of utmost importance to address the investigation [5] (Fig. 9.1).

A leading cause of arrhythmic SCD without morphological substrate is long QT (LQT) syndrome, a genetically determined autosomal or recessive disease, characterized by a long QT interval (>450 msec) (Fig. 9.2) due to prolonged repolarization of the working myocardium, which causes an electrical vulnerability with possible onset of life-threatening arrhythmias, including torsades de pointes and ventricular fibrillation [8–11]. There are three main forms of LQT syndrome: LQT1 and LQT2 are mostly related to loss of function mutations in genes encoding potassium channel, whereas LQT3 is due to mutations of genes encoding sodium channel, namely SCN5A, the same gene involved in Brugada syndrome and Lenegre's disease with AV block. Cardiac arrest occurs usually during exercise in LQT1, emotion in LQT2, and sleep in LQT3 [8].

The short QT syndrome, a Mendelian disorder with autosomal dominant pattern of inheritance, is much rarer than the LQT syndrome and is characterized by a QT interval shorter than 320 msec [12]. It has been linked to potassium gene mutations, with gain of function and shortening of the action potential. SCD occurs mostly during sleep.

Brugada (or Martini–Nava–Thiene) syndrome is an autosomal dominant inherited disorder characterized mostly by loss of function mutations of SCN5A sodium channel gene and featured by a nonischemic ST segment elevation at 12-lead ECG [13, 14]. Only 20 % of cases were found so far to have a genetic basis, whereas the remaining are still unexplained at molecular level [15, 16]. It is still a matter of debate whether hearts of patients dying suddenly with Brugada syndrome are structurally normal or present subtle changes (i.e., concealed structural cardiomyopathy), mimicking arrhythmogenic cardiomyopathy [13, 17, 18].

Catecholaminergic polymorphic ventricular tachycardia (CPVT) is a heredofamilial disorder of the calcium homeostasis [19, 20]. The defect involves the Ca++ uptake and release from the smooth sarcoplasmic reticulum, accounting for electromechanical coupling. The autosomal dominant form is characterized by a mutation of the ryanodine receptor 2 gene, which causes a Ca++ excessive release into the cytosol, impairing the sodium–calcium exchange at the level of the sarcolemma [20–23]. This interferes with myocyte repolarization and may trigger life-threatening arrhythmias. The autosomal recessive form is due to mutations of calsequestrin 2 gene, which regulates the reuptake of the calcium into the sarcoplasmic reticulum [24, 25].

The onset of life-threatening ventricular arrhythmias is rate dependent. When, during effort or emotion, the heart rate exceeds 120–125 bpm, onset of polymorphic ventricular arrhythmias and even ventricular fibrillation may occur. Stress test ECG is a fundamental tool to clinically unmask the disorder (Fig. 9.3) [26].

Many cases of SCD without substrate still remain unexplained, even after a thorough investigation of genes known to be related to the abovementioned syndromes. They still belong to the category of idiopathic ventricular fibrillation. Dysfunction of the Purkinje fibers has been advanced, with early repolarization wave at the ECG (the so-called Haissaguerre syndrome) [27].

With the genome-wide investigation technique, it is foreseeable that eventually a genetic explanation will be found in many other cases of "mors sine materia." However, after the initial emphasis, caution is needed due to the difficult interpretation of the pathogenic significance of gene mutations in the absence of family history and cascade genetic screening [28–32].

© Springer-Verlag Milan 2016
G. Thiene et al., *Sudden Cardiac Death in the Young and Athletes: Text Atlas of Pathology and Clinical Correlates*,
DOI 10.1007/978-88-470-5776-0_9

9.1   Image Gallery

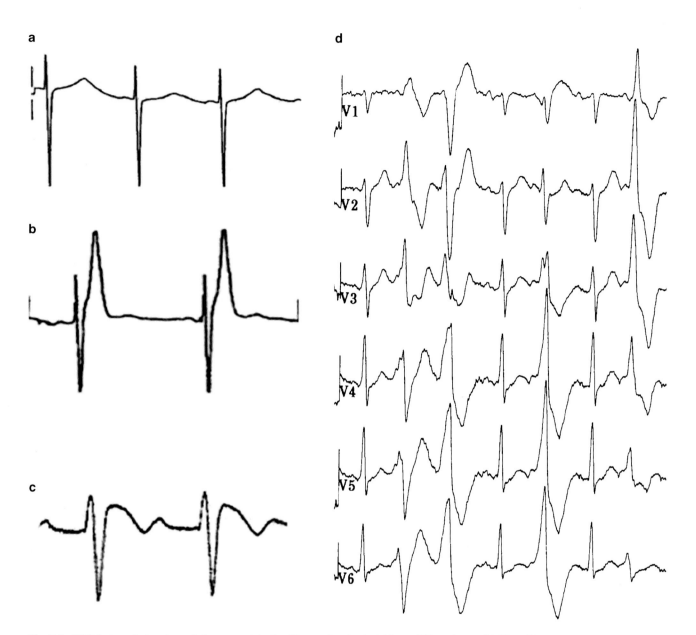

Fig. 9.1 ECG features in ion channel diseases at risk of sudden cardiac death. (**a**) Long QT syndrome. (**b**) Short QT syndrome. (**c**) Brugada syndrome. (**d**) Catecholaminergic polymorphic ventricular tachycardia (stress test ECG)

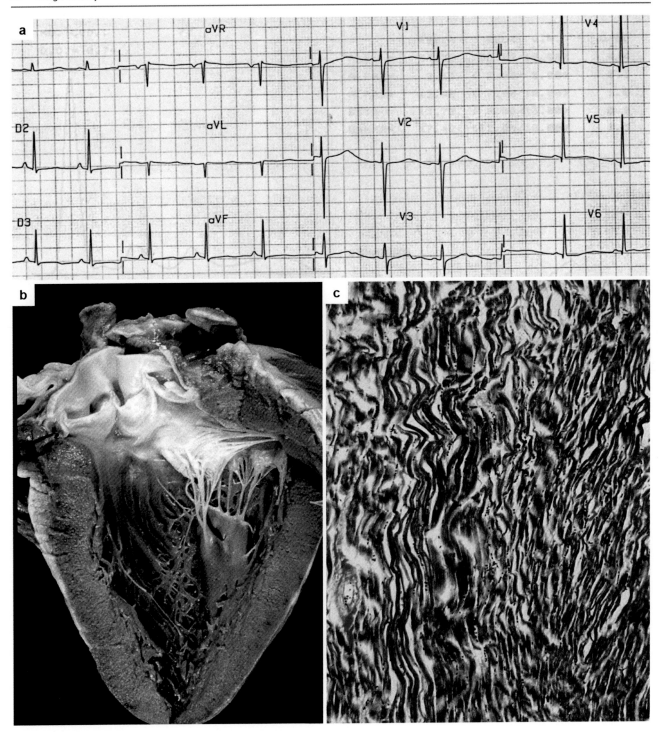

Fig. 9.2 Arrhythmic sudden cardiac death with normal heart in a 21-year-old young man while swimming. (a) 12-lead ECG showing the prolonged QT interval (QTc = 480 msec). (b) Grossly normal heart at autopsy. (c) Histology of the left ventricular myocardium reveals only waviness of the myofibers following cardiac arrest (Heidenhain trichrome)

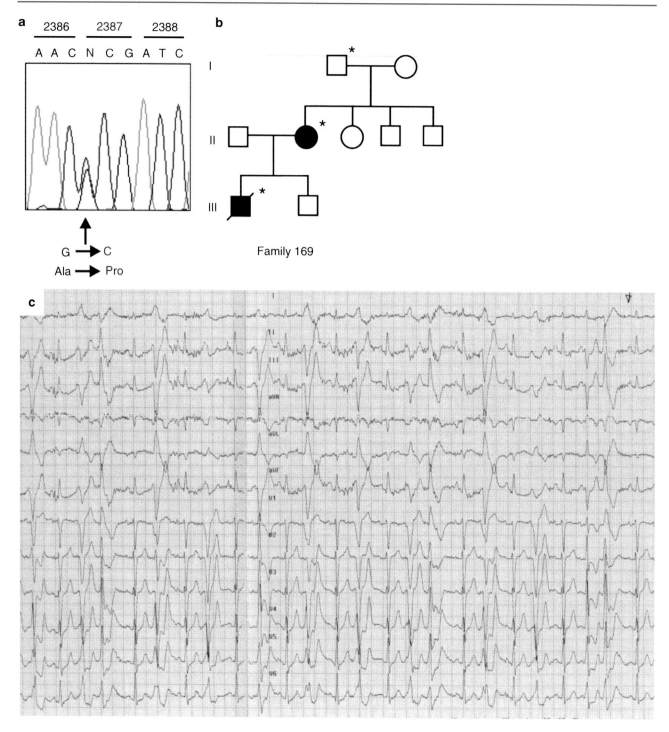

Fig. 9.3 Arrhythmic sudden cardiac death with normal heart in a 16-year-old boy on emotion. (**a**) Genetic analysis, performed at post-mortem, of the DNA extracted from frozen spleen sample discovered a missense mutation (c.7160 G>C) at exon 47 of the ryanodine receptor 2 gene, accounting for amino acid change Ala2387Pro. (**b**) By extending the investigation to the family members, genetic screening revealed that the mother and the maternal grandfather carried the same mutation. (**c**) Polymorphous ventricular arrhythmias in the affected mother, triggered during stress test; (*asterisc*) indicates gene mutation carrier; *black symbol* indicates family member clinically affected by catecholaminergic polymorphic ventricular tachycardia

References

1. Thiene G, Carturan E, Corrado D, Basso C. Prevention of sudden cardiac death in the young and in athletes: dream or reality? Cardiovasc Pathol. 2010;19:207–17.

2. Thiene G. Sudden cardiac death and cardiovascular pathology: from anatomic theater to double helix. Am J Cardiol. 2014; 114:1930–6.

3. Corrado D, Basso C, Thiene G. Sudden cardiac death in young people with apparently normal heart. Cardiovasc Res. 2001;50: 399–408.

4. Basso C, Carturan E, Pilichou K, Rizzo S, Corrado D, Thiene G. Sudden cardiac death with normal heart: molecular autopsy. Cardiovasc Pathol. 2010;19:321–5.

5. Basso C, Burke M, Fornes P, Gallagher PJ, de Gouveia RH, Sheppard M, Thiene G, van der Wal A, Association for European Cardiovascular Pathology. Guidelines for autopsy investigation of sudden cardiac death. Virchows Arch. 2008;452:11–8.

6. Thiene G, Corrado D, Basso C. Cardiomyopathies: is it time for a molecular classification? Eur Heart J. 2004;25:1772–5.

7. Maron BJ, Towbin JA, Thiene G, Antzelevitch C, Corrado D, Arnett D, Moss AJ, Seidman CE, Young JB. Contemporary definitions and classification of the cardiomyopathies: an American Heart Association Scientific Statement from the Council on Clinical Cardiology, Heart Failure and Transplantation Committee; Quality of Care and Outcomes Research and Functional Genomics and Translational Biology Interdisciplinary Working Groups; and Council on Epidemiology and Prevention. Circulation. 2006;113:1807–16.

8. Priori SG, Schwartz PJ, Napolitano C, Bloise R, Ronchetti E, Grillo M, Vicentini A, Spazzolini C, Nastoli J, Bottelli G, Folli R, Cappelletti D. Risk stratification in the long-QT syndrome. N Engl J Med. 2003;348:1866–74.

9. Curran ME, Splawski I, Timothy KW, Vincent GM, Green ED, Keating MT. A molecular basis for cardiac arrhythmia: HERG mutations cause long QT syndrome. Cell. 1995;80:795–803.

10. Wang Q, Curran ME, Splawski I, Burn TC, Millholland JM, VanRaay TJ, Shen J, Timothy KW, Vincent GM, de Jager T, Schwartz PJ, Towbin JA, Moss AJ, Atkinson DL, Landes GM, Connors TD, Keating MT. Positional cloning of a novel potassium channel gene: KvLQT1 mutations cause cardiac arrhythmias. Nat Genet. 1996;12:17–23.

11. Wang Q, Shen J, Splawski I, Atkinson D, Li Z, Robinson JL, Moss AJ, Towbin JA, Keating MT. SCN5A mutations associated with an inherited cardiac arrhythmia, long QT syndrome. Cell. 1995;80:805–11.

12. Patel C, Yan GX, Antzelevitch C. Short QT syndrome: from bench to bedside. Circ Arrhythm Electrophysiol. 2010;3:401–8.

13. Martini B, Nava A, Thiene G, Buja GF, Canciani B, Scognamiglio R, Daliento L, Dalla Volta S. Ventricular fibrillation without apparent heart disease: description of six cases. Am Heart J. 1989;118: 1203–9.

14. Brugada P, Brugada J. Right bundle branch block, persistent ST segment elevation and sudden cardiac death: a distinct clinical and electrocardiographic syndrome. J Am Coll Cardiol. 1992;20: 1391–6.

15. Brugada P, Brugada J, Roy D. Brugada syndrome 1992–2012: 20 years of scientific excitement, and more. Eur Heart J. 2013; 34:3610–5.

16. Li A, Behr ER. Brugada syndrome: an update. Future Cardiol. 2013;9:253–71.

17. Corrado D, Basso C, Buja G, Nava A, Rossi L, Thiene G. Right bundle branch block, right precordial st-segment elevation, and sudden death in young people. Circulation. 2001;103:710–7.

18. Corrado D, Nava A, Buja G, Martini B, Fasoli G, Oselladore L, Turrini P, Thiene G. Familial cardiomyopathy underlies syndrome of right bundle branch block, ST segment elevation and sudden death. J Am Coll Cardiol. 1996;27:443–8.

19. Leenhardt A, Lucet V, Denjoy I, Grau F, Ngoc DD, Coumel P. Catecholaminergic polymorphic ventricular tachycardia in children. A 7-year follow-up of 21 patients. Circulation. 1995;91: 1512–9.

20. Tiso N, Stephan DA, Nava A, Bagattin A, Devaney JM, Stanchi F, Larderet G, Brahmbhatt B, Brown K, Bauce B, Muriago M, Basso C, Thiene G, Danieli GA, Rampazzo A. Identification of mutations in the cardiac ryanodine receptor gene in families affected with arrhythmogenic right ventricular cardiomyopathy type 2 (ARVD2). Hum Mol Genet. 2001;10:189–94.

21. Priori SG, Napolitano C, Tiso N, Memmi M, Vignati G, Bloise R, Sorrentino V, Danieli GA. Mutations in the cardiac ryanodine receptor gene (hRyR2) underlie catecholaminergic polymorphic ventricular tachycardia. Circulation. 2001;103:196–200.

22. Priori SG, Napolitano C, Memmi M, Colombi B, Drago F, Gasparini M, DeSimone L, Coltorti F, Bloise R, Keegan R, Cruz Filho FE, Vignati G, Benatar A, DeLogu A. Clinical and molecular characterization of patients with catecholaminergic polymorphic ventricular tachycardia. Circulation. 2002;106:69–74.

23. van der Werf C, Wilde AA. Catecholaminergic polymorphic ventricular tachycardia: from bench to bedside. Heart. 2013;99: 497–504.

24. Lahat H, Pras E, Olender T, Avidan N, Ben-Asher E, Man O, Levy-Nissenbaum E, Khoury A, Lorber A, Goldman B, Lancet D, Eldar M. A missense mutation in a highly conserved region of CASQ2 is associated with autosomal recessive catecholamine-induced polymorphic ventricular tachycardia in Bedouin families from Israel. Am J Hum Genet. 2001;69:1378–84.

25. Postma AV, Denjoy I, Hoorntje TM, Lupoglazoff JM, Da Costa A, Sebillon P, Mannens MM, Wilde AA, Guicheney P. Absence of calsequestrin 2 causes severe forms of catecholaminergic polymorphic ventricular tachycardia. Circ Res. 2002;91:e21–6.

26. Bauce B, Rampazzo A, Basso C, Bagattin A, Daliento L, Tiso N, Turrini P, Thiene G, Danieli GA, Nava A. Screening for ryanodine receptor type 2 mutations in families with effort-induced polymorphic ventricular arrhythmias and sudden death: early diagnosis of asymptomatic carriers. J Am Coll Cardiol. 2002;40:341–9.

27. Haïssaguerre M, Derval N, Sacher F, Jesel L, Deisenhofer I, de Roy L, Pasquié JL, Nogami A, Babuty D, Yli-Mayry S, De Chillou C, Scanu P, Mabo P, Matsuo S, Probst V, Le Scouarnec S, Defaye P, Schlaepfer J, Rostock T, Lacroix D, Lamaison D, Lavergne T, Aizawa Y, Englund A, Anselme F, O'Neill M, Hocini M, Lim KT, Knecht S, Veenhuyzen GD, Bordachar P, Chauvin M, Jais P, Coureau G, Chene G, Klein GJ, Clémenty J. Sudden cardiac arrest associated with early repolarization. N Engl J Med. 2008;358: 2016–23.

28. Semsarian C, Ingles J, Wilde AA. Sudden cardiac death in the young: the molecular autopsy and a practical approach to surviving relatives. Eur Heart J. 2015;36:1290–6.

29. Tester DJ, Medeiros-Domingo A, Will ML, Haglund CM, Ackerman MJ. Cardiac channel molecular autopsy: insights from 173 consecutive cases of autopsy-negative sudden unexplained death referred for postmortem genetic testing. Mayo Clin Proc. 2012;87:524–39.

30. Tester DJ, Ackerman MJ. Postmortem long QT syndrome genetic testing for sudden unexplained death in the young. J Am Coll Cardiol. 2007;49:240–6.

31. Tester DJ, Ackerman MJ. The role of molecular autopsy in unexplained sudden cardiac death. Curr Opin Cardiol. 2006;21:166–72.

32. Priori SG, Wilde AA, Horie M, Cho Y, Behr ER, Berul C, Blom N, Brugada J, Chiang CE, Huikuri H, Kannankeril P, Krahn A, Leenhardt A, Moss A, Schwartz PJ, Shimizu W, Tomaselli G, Tracy C. Executive summary: HRS/EHRA/APHRS expert consensus statement on the diagnosis and management of patients with inherited primary arrhythmia syndromes. Heart Rhythm. 2013;10: e85–108.

How to Study Sudden Death at Autopsy: Protocol of Investigation

Since SD, especially in the young, is frequently the first and last symptom of an underlying disease, the autopsy is the only way to establish the cause. Thus, it should be regularly carried out, not only for the right of the family and community to have an explanation of this dramatic event but also for the implications on the surviving relatives [1]. About 30–40 % of SDs are indeed ascribable to genetically determined, transmissible morbid entities, mostly with an autosomal dominant pattern of inheritance, so that 50 % of the first-degree relatives are potentially affected ("carriers") of the mutation and exposed at risk [1–5].

As emphasized in the guidelines of the Association for European Cardiovascular Pathology, the role of the autopsy is to establish [1]:

(a) Whether the death is attributable to natural or unnatural causes and, if natural, to a cardiac or extracardiac disease
(b) The nature of the cardiac disease and whether the mechanism was arrhythmic or mechanical
(c) Whether the cardiac condition, causing SD, may be inherited, requiring screening and counseling of the next of kin
(d) If toxic or illicit drug abuse is involved and if other unnatural deaths played a role

10.1 Clinical Information Relevant to Autopsy

Gathering the relevant clinical information is mandatory for a clinicopathologic correlation [1]:

- Age, gender, occupation, and lifestyle (alcohol, tabagism, etc.)

- Circumstances of death: witnessed or unwitnessed, any suspicious circumstances (carbon monoxide, violence, traffic accident, electrical burst, etc.), and ECG tracing recorded during resuscitation
- Family history, especially cardiac: ischemic heart disease, premature SD, arrhythmias, and inherited arrhythmic disorders
- Medical history: general health status, previous significant illnesses (syncope, epilepsy, chest pain, palpitations particularly during exercise, etc.), previous surgical or nonsurgical interventions (pacemaker, implantable cardioverter defibrillator-ICD, etc.), ECG tracings and chest X-rays, echo, and any laboratory findings (lipid profiles, serum enzymes and troponin measurements, medication, etc.)

10.2 External Examination of the Body

- Establish body weight and height (to correlate with heart weight and wall thickness).
- Check for recent intravenous access, intubation, ECG pads, defibrillator and electrical burns, drain sites, and traumatic lesions.
- Check for ICD/pacemaker; if in situ, see MDA Safety Notice 2002 for safe removal and interrogation.

10.3 Sequential Approach to Establish the Causes of Sudden Death through Full Autopsy Technique

Noncardiac causes of sudden death should be first excluded [1]. Any natural sudden death can be considered cardiac in origin after the exclusion of noncardiac causes. Thus, a full

© Springer-Verlag Milan 2016
G. Thiene et al., *Sudden Cardiac Death in the Young and Athletes: Text Atlas of Pathology and Clinical Correlates*,
DOI 10.1007/978-88-470-5776-0_10

autopsy with sequential approach should be always performed to rule out common and uncommon extracardiac causes of SD:

- Cerebral (subarachnoid or intracerebral hemorrhage, etc.)
- Respiratory (allergic, asthma, anaphylaxis, etc.)
- Acute hemorrhagic shock (ruptured aortic aneurysm, gastrointestinal hemorrhage, etc.)
- Septic shock (Waterhouse–Friderichsen syndrome, etc.)

10.4 Search for the Cardiac Culprit: The Standard Gross Examination

The search for the cardiac culprit should address the vital components of the heart [1]: great arteries, coronary arteries, myocardium, valves, and conduction system.

The standard gross examination of the heart should be carried out as follows:

1. Check the pericardium, open and explore the pericardial cavity (Fig. 10.1).
2. Check the great arteries before transecting them, 3 cm above the aortic and pulmonary valves, and open the pulmonary artery and bifurcation (Fig. 10.2).
3. Check and transect the pulmonary veins. Transect the superior vena cava 2 cm above the point where the crista terminalis meets the superior vena cava (sulcus terminalis), to preserve the sinus node. Transect the inferior vena cava close to the diaphragm.
4. Open the right atrium from the inferior vena cava to the apex of the right atrial appendage. Open the left atrium between the pulmonary veins and then to the atrial appendage (Fig. 10.3).
5. Inspect the atrial cavities and the interatrial septum, and determine whether the foramen ovale is patent. Examine the mitral and tricuspid valves (or valve prostheses) and check the integrity of the papillary muscles and chordae tendineae.
6. Inspect the aorta, the pulmonary artery, and the aortic and pulmonary valves (or valve prosthesis).
7. Then the coronary arteries are grossly investigated as follows:
   (a) Examine the size, shape, position, number, and patency of the coronary ostia (Fig. 10.4).
   (b) Assess the size, course, and "dominance" of the major epicardial arteries.
   (c) Make multiple transverse cuts at 3 mm intervals along the course of the main epicardial arteries and branches, such as the diagonal and obtuse marginal ones, and check patency (Figs. 10.5 and 10.6).
   (d) Heavily calcified coronary arteries have sometimes to be opened adequately with sharp scissors. If this

is not possible, they should be removed intact, decalcified, and opened transversely.
   (e) Coronary artery segments containing metallic stents should be referred intact to labs with facilities for resin embedding and subsequent processing and sectioning.
   (f) Coronary artery bypass grafts (saphenous veins, internal mammary arteries, radial arteries, etc.) should be carefully examined with transverse cuts. The proximal and distal anastomoses should be examined with particular care.
8. Make a complete transverse (short-axis) cut of the heart at the midventricular level and then parallel slices of ventricles at 1 cm intervals toward the apex (Fig. 10.7), and assess these slices carefully for thickness of the walls and size of the cavities, as well as abnormalities of the myocardium.
9. Once emptied of blood, make the following measurements:
   - Total heart weight (against tables of normal weights by age, gender, and body weight).
   - Heart wall thickness: inspect the endocardium and measure thickness of the mid-cavity free wall of the left ventricle, right ventricle, and septum (excluding trabeculae), against tables of normal thickness by age, gender, and body weight.
   - Heart dimensions: the transverse size is best calculated as the distance from the obtuse to the acute margin in the posterior AV sulcus. The longitudinal size is obtained from a measurement of the distance between the crux cordis and the apex of the heart on the posterior aspect.
10. Open the basal half of the heart along the blood flow direction and complete the examination of atrial and ventricular septa, AV valves, ventricular inflows and outflows, and semilunar valves (Fig. 10.8). In case of ECG-documented ventricular preexcitation, the AV rings should be maintained intact.

10.5 Standard Histological Examination of the Heart

- Coronary arteries: in the setting of coronary artery disease, the severe focal lesions should be sampled for histology in labeled blocks and stained routinely with hematoxylin-eosin and a connective tissue stain (elastic Weigert–van Gieson, trichrome, or Sirius red). Special stains and immunohistochemistry should be performed as deemed necessary.
- Myocardium: take mapped labeled blocks from a representative transverse slice of the ventricles to include the free wall of the left ventricle (anterior, lateral, and

posterior), the ventricular septum (anterior and posterior), the free wall of the right ventricle (anterior, lateral, and posterior) (Fig. 10.9), right ventricular outflow tract (Fig. 10.10), and one block from each atria.

In addition, any area with significant macroscopic abnormalities should be sampled. Hematoxylin-eosin and a connective tissue stain are standard. Special stains and immunohistochemistry should be performed as required.

- Other cardiac samples (such as valve tissue, pericardium, and aorta) as indicated.

Of course, histology should be carried out on samples from any other organ.

10.6 Ultrastructural Examination

If there is the suspicion of rare cardiomyopathies (mitochondrial, storage, infiltrative, etc.), a small sample of myocardium (1 mm³) should be fixed in 2,5 % glutaraldehyde for electron microscopy examination.

10.7 Histologic Study of the Conduction System

If the clinical history and ECG tracing suggest an electrical conduction abnormality, investigation of the conduction system through serial sections technique should be performed, removing and embedding in paraffin two blocks with sinoatrial and septal AV junctions, respectively (Fig. 10.11).

In case of ECG-proven Wolff–Parkinson–White syndrome, the serial section investigation should be extended to the lateral left and right rings in search of accessory pathways. Precise interpretation of the ECG facilitates the topographic identification of the abnormal conduction pathway, pointing where to remove the tissue block and make histologic serial sectioning (Fig. 10.12).

10.8 Molecular Autopsy

Molecular autopsy in case of SD aims to study DNA/RNA in the setting of suspected myocarditis or structural and nonstructural genetically determined heart disease [1].

In both cases, 10 ml of EDTA blood and 5 g of myocardium (from the left ventricular free wall) (Fig. 10.13) and spleen and/or liver should be taken, frozen, and stored at −80 °C or alternatively stored in RNA later at 4 °C for up to 2 weeks and nucleic acid extraction accomplished through thermocycler.

From fresh tissue, RNA later, autoptic blood in EDTA or frozen tissue, nucleic acid extraction, and gene sequencing can be carried out with success up to 100 % of cases, even when amplicon length is greater than 300 bp.

From formalin-fixed and paraffin-embedded tissue, nucleic acid extraction is successful in up to 85 % of cases and only when amplicon length is less than 300 bp (viruses, for instance).

These aspects will be discussed more in detail in Chap. 11.

10.9 Toxicological Investigation

In case of suspicion, especially in unwitnessed or SD victims found dead at bed, heart blood (25 ml), peripheral blood from femoral veins (10 ml), urine (30–50 ml), or bile (20–30 ml) if urine is not available, should be stored at 4° and undergo a toxicological analysis.

A lock of hair (100–200 mg) should be cut from the back head or from the pubes. The toxicological analysis should be quantitative and performed in certified referral laboratories.

10.10 Formulation of a Diagnosis, with Clinicopathologic Correlates and Epicrisis

In the majority of SD cases, a clear pathological cause can be identified already at gross and histological investigation, albeit with varying degrees of confidence [1].

However, it is important to recognize that different degrees of certainty exist in defining the cause–effect relationship between the observed cardiovascular substrate and the SCD event.

The commonest substrates of SCD are classified as certain, highly probable, or uncertain (Table 10.1). Acute occlusive coronary thrombosis, embolism or dissection, cardiac tamponade due to aortic rupture (Fig. 10.1), and pulmonary thromboembolism (Fig. 10.2) should be considered certain. When, in case of coronary artery atherosclerosis, the coronary stenosis exceeds 75 % degree (critical stenosis), in the absence of other explanation, the cause may be considered highly probable [5].

Some coronary artery congenital anomalies, like left circumflex arterial branch from the right coronary artery/aortic sinus and myocardial bridge, should be regarded as uncertain substrates, since these conditions may be a variant of normal. In these circumstances, nonstructural arrhythmic diseases should be always investigated in the personal and family history. Within the improbable and uncertain categories, each case should be considered on its individual merits, and the clinical history and the circumstances of death may influence the decision-making process.

Finally, there are diagnostic "gray zones" in which the border between physiological and pathological changes is poorly defined. This is the case of fatty tissue of the right ventricular free wall vs. arrhythmogenic cardiomyopathy, athlete's heart vs. hypertrophic cardiomyopathy, myocardial disarray in the absence of hypertrophy vs. hypertrophic cardiomyopathy without hypertrophy, and focal inflammatory infiltrates vs. borderline myocarditis (Table 10.2) [1].

In conclusion, wherever possible, the most likely underlying cause should be stated and the need for familial clinical screening and genetic analysis clearly indicated.

10.11   Final Recommendations

The best practice is that the entire heart is retained and sent to specialized centers. The referring pathologist should complete standard gross examination of the specimen, make a transverse apical section, and empty the heart of blood. Tissue, blood, and other fluids for molecular pathology and toxicology should be taken, before fixing the heart in formalin 10 %. It is strongly recommended the heart be preserved for leaving the possibility of other gross revisitation and histologic sampling. If the heart cannot be retained, it is essential that extensive photographic documentation is made, indicating where individual blocks are taken.

Table 10.1 The diagnosis of sudden cardiac death at autopsy may be classified as certain, highly probable, and uncertain

Certain	Highly probable	Uncertain
Massive pulmonary embolism	Stable atherosclerotic plaque with luminal stenosis >75 %, with or without healed myocardial infarction	Minor anomalies of the coronary arteries from the aorta (RCA from the left sinus, LCA from the right without inter-arterial course, high take-off from the tubular portion, LCX originating from the right sinus or RCA, coronary ostia plication, fibromuscular dysplasia, intramural small vessel disease)
Hemopericardium due to aortic or cardiac rupture	Anomalous origin of the LCA from the right sinus and inter-arterial course	Intramyocardial course of a coronary artery (myocardial bridge)
Mitral valve papillary muscle or chordae tendineae rupture with acute mitral valve incompetence and pulmonary edema	Cardiomyopathies (hypertrophic, arrhythmogenic, dilated, others)	Focal myocarditis, hypertensive heart disease, idiopathic left ventricular hypertrophy
Acute coronary occlusion due to thrombosis, dissection, or embolism	Myxoid degeneration of the mitral valve with prolapse, with atrial dilatation or left ventricular hypertrophy and intact chordae	Myxoid degeneration of the mitral valve with prolapse, without atrial dilatation or left ventricular hypertrophy and intact chordae
Anomalous origin of the coronary artery from the pulmonary trunk	Aortic stenosis with left ventricular hypertrophy	Dystrophic calcification of the membranous septum (±mitral annulus/aortic valve)
Neoplasm/thrombus obstructing the valve orifice	ECG-documented ventricular preexcitation (Wolff–Parkinson–White syndrome, Lown–Ganong–Levine syndrome)	Atrial septum lipoma
Thrombotic block of the valve prosthesis	ECG-documented sinoatrial or AV block	AV node cystic tumor without ECG evidence of AV block, conducting system disease without ECG documentation
Laceration/dehiscence/poppet escape of the valve prosthesis with acute valve incompetence	Congenital heart diseases, operated	Congenital heart diseases, unoperated, with or without Eisenmenger syndrome
Massive acute myocarditis		

From Basso et al. [1]. *AV* atrioventricular; *LCA* left coronary artery; *LCX* left circumflex; *RCA* right coronary artery

Table 10.2 Gray zone conditions which may be misinterpreted as pathological changes responsible of sudden cardiac death

Physiological change	Pathological change
Fatty infiltration of the right ventricular wall	Arrhythmogenic cardiomyopathy
Exercise-induced left ventricular hypertrophy (athlete's heart)	Hypertrophic cardiomyopathy
Focal myocardial disarray without hypertrophy	Hypertrophic cardiomyopathy without hypertrophy
Scattered inflammatory foci with or without small foci of fibrosis	Borderline/focal myocarditis

From Basso et al. [1]

10.12   Image Gallery

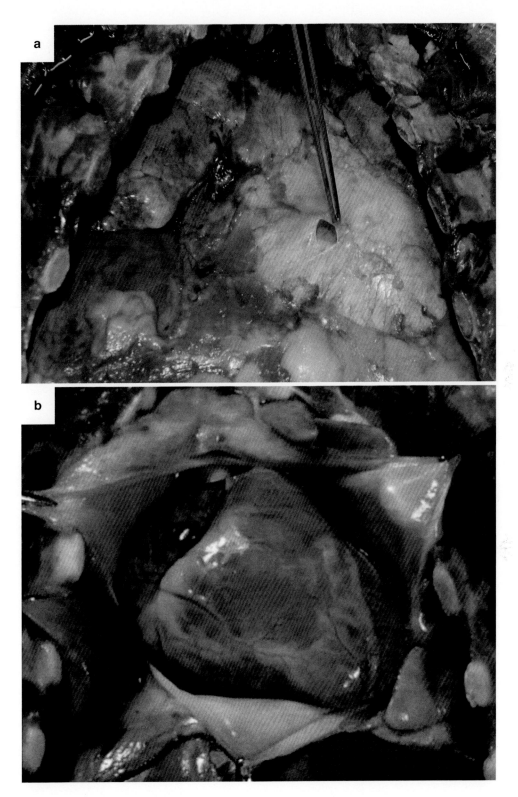

Fig. 10.1 Check from outside (**a**) and open the pericardial cavity (**b**) to search for cardiac tamponade

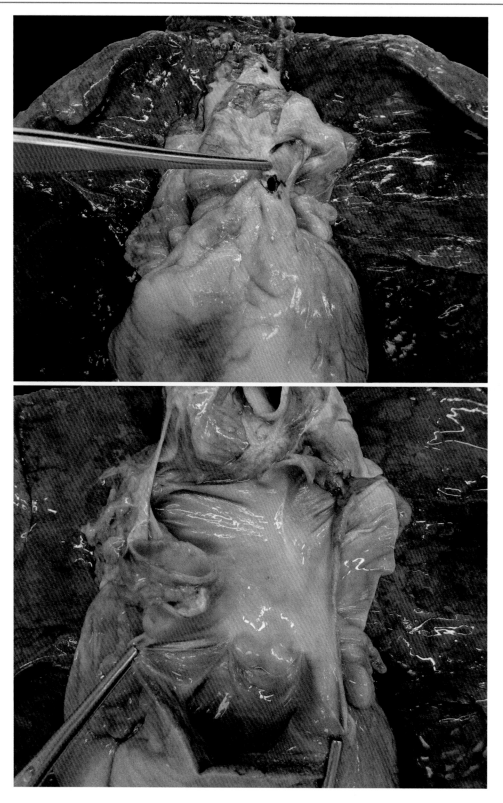

Fig. 10.2 Open the pulmonary artery (a) and extend longitudinally along the main trunk and bifurcation (b), up to the pulmonary hilus bilaterally, to search for thromboembolism

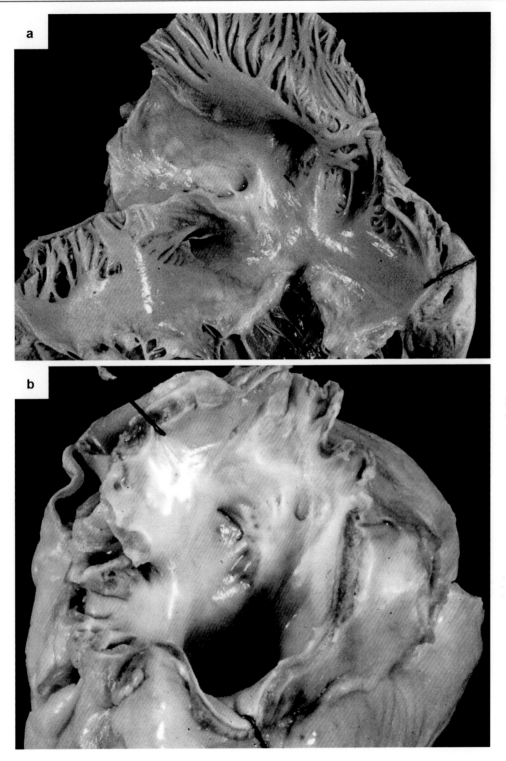

Fig. 10.3 Opening of the atria to explore the cavities and the atrioventricular valves. (**a**) The right atrium is open with a cut from the inferior vena cava up to the right atrial appendage (avoid an inferior-to-superior vena cava cut, not to section the crista terminalis and sinus node). (**b**) The left atrium is open with a cut from a pulmonary vein to the contralateral one and then complete with an opening of the left atrial appendage up to the distal part

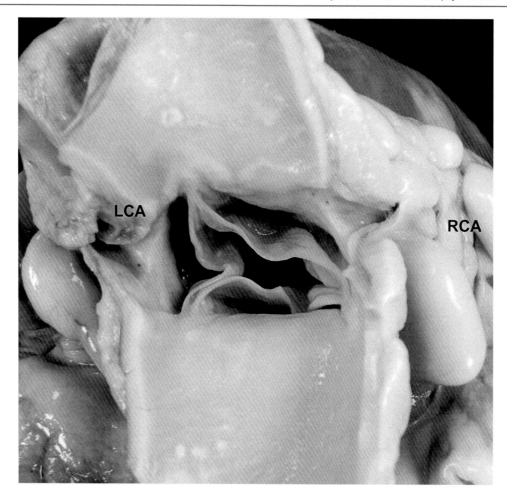

Fig. 10.4 After a transection of the aorta 3 cm above the aortic valve, inspection of the aortic valve and of the coronary ostia location in the proper aortic sinus (LCA = left coronary artery; RCA = right coronary artery)

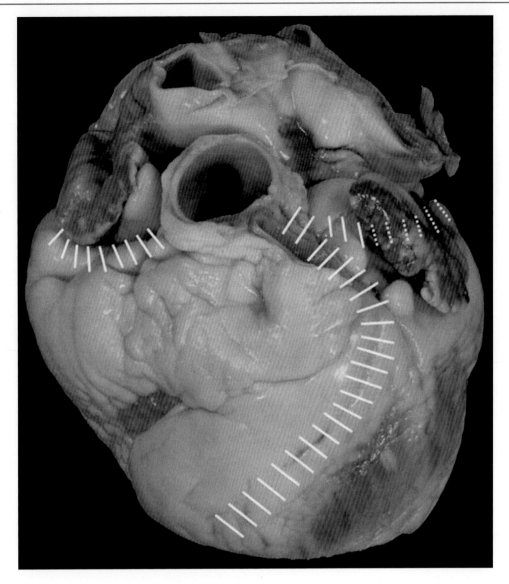

Fig. 10.5 Schematic representation of serial cross sectioning of the subepicardial coronary artery tree

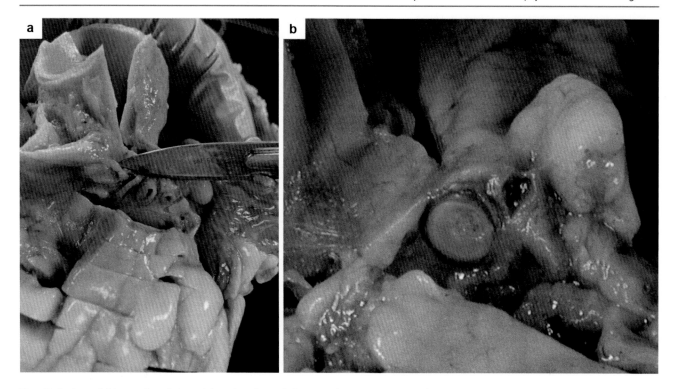

Fig. 10.6 A careful inspection of the serial sections is needed not to miss any coronary lesion. (**a**) Nonobstructive atherosclerotic plaque of the first tract of the left anterior descending coronary artery. (**b**) Transverse cut of the first tract appears occluded by thrombosis

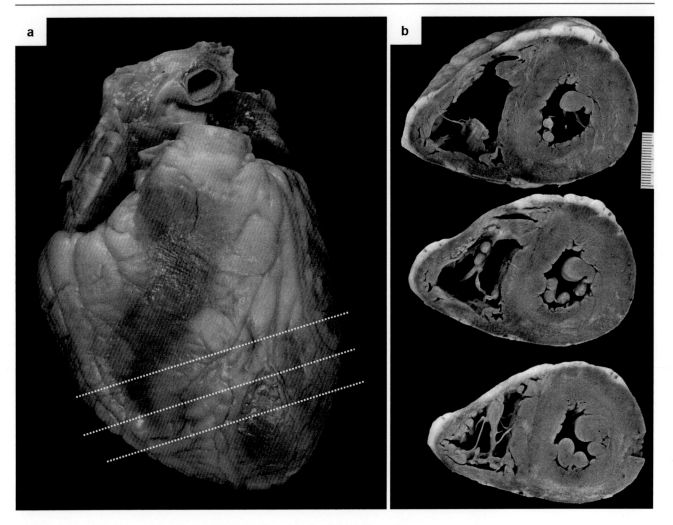

Fig. 10.7 Short-axis cross sectioning of the heart specimen from midventricular to apical levels. (**a**) Gross view of the specimen before cross sectioning. (**b**) Transverse sections of the heart at the three different levels as represented in (**a**)

Fig. 10.8 Opening of the
ventricular cavities along the
blood flow direction. (**a**) Right
ventricular inflow–outflow.
(**b**) Left ventricular
inflow–outflow

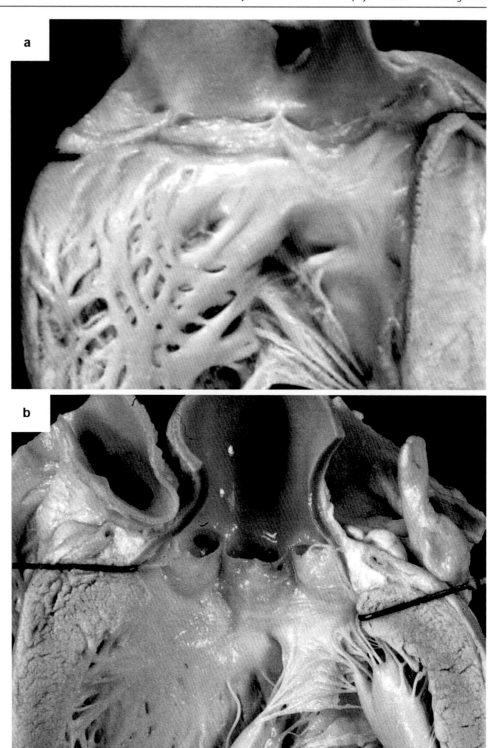

Fig. 10.9 Sampling of the myocardium with several transmural blocks, circumferentially in the entire transverse section of the heart, along the left ventricle, septum, and right ventricle

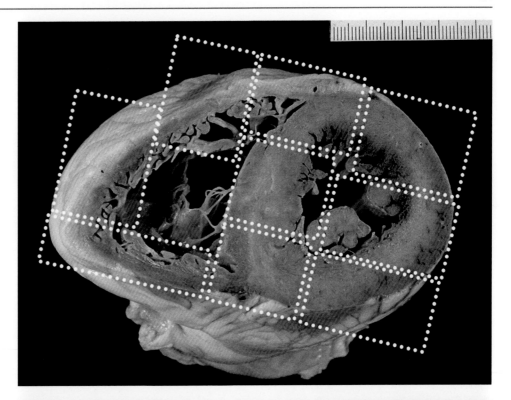

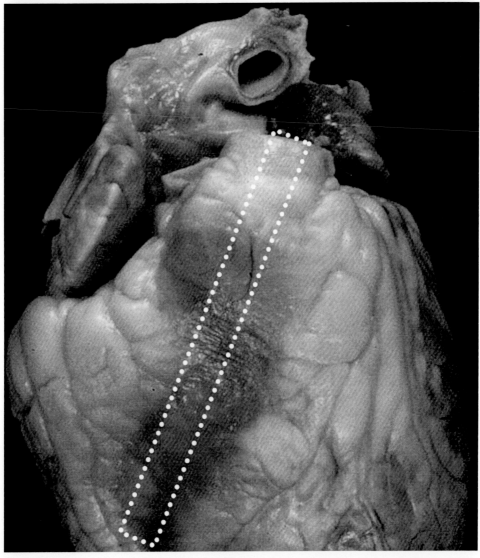

Fig. 10.10 An additional sampling of the right ventricular outflow tract can be also taken

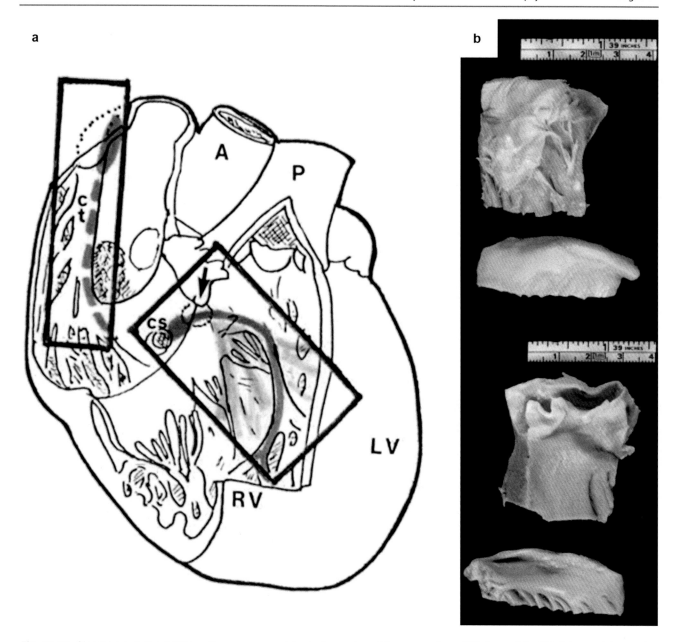

Fig. 10.11 Sinoatrial and septal AV junctions are removed in single blocks, embedded in paraffin and submitted to serial sectioning. (**a**) Drawing of the blocks to be sampled, including the sinus node and the atrioventricular node. (**b**) Resulting tissue blocks; *A* aorta; *P* pulmonary artery; *CS* coronary sinus; *LV* left ventricle; *RV* right ventricle; *ct* crista terminalis; *arrow* indicated membranous septum (original drawing by Professor Lino Rossi)

Fig. 10.12 Ventricular preexcitation due to an accessory pathway localized in the right AV ring causing arrhythmic sudden cardiac death in a 26-year-old man. (**a**) The ECG with the delta wave of preexcitation indicates the accessory pathway in the right AV ring. (**b**) View of the right atrium and ventricle, with drawing of the location of the accessory pathway along the tricuspid valve found at histology

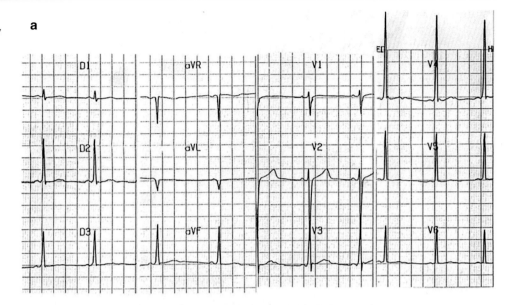

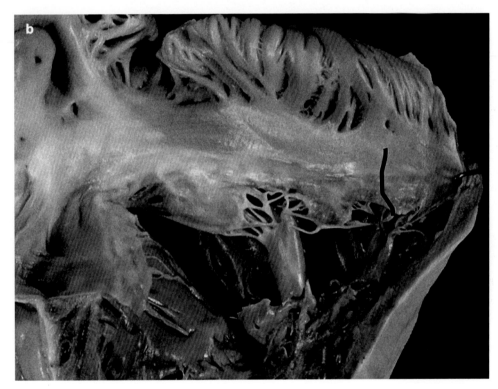

Fig. 10.13 Block of myocardium is taken from the left ventricle at autopsy and then frozen and stored at −80°, to be submitted for possible molecular investigations

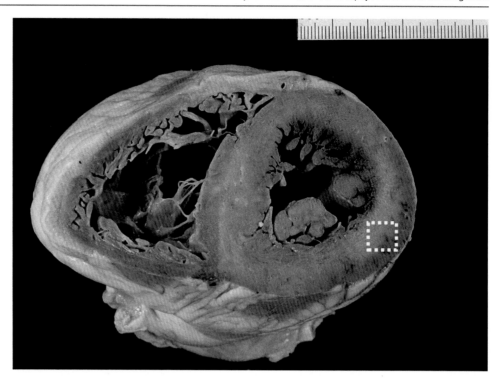

References

1. Basso C, Burke M, Fornes P, Gallagher PJ, de Gouveia RH, Sheppard M, Thiene G, van der Wal A, Association for European Cardiovascular Pathology. Guidelines for autopsy investigation of sudden cardiac death. Virchows Arch. 2008;452:11–8.
2. Thiene G. Sudden cardiac death and cardiovascular pathology: from anatomic theater to double helix. Am J Cardiol. 2014;114:1930–6.
3. Thiene G, Carturan E, Corrado D, Basso C. Prevention of sudden cardiac death in the young and in athletes: dream or reality? Cardiovasc Pathol. 2010;19:207–17.
4. Basso C, Calabrese F, Corrado D, Thiene G. Postmortem diagnosis in sudden cardiac death victims: macroscopic, microscopic and molecular findings. Cardiovasc Res. 2001;50:290–330.
5. Basso C, Carturan E, Pilichou K, Rizzo S, Corrado D, Thiene G. Sudden cardiac death with normal heart: molecular autopsy. Cardiovasc Pathol. 2010;19:321–5.

Molecular autopsy in case of SCD aims to investigate DNA/RNA into two different settings: (a) myocarditis, for the detection of infective agents, mainly DNA and RNA cardiotropic viruses and (b) structural and nonstructural genetically determined heart diseases, for the search of pathogenic gene mutations [1, 2].

For this reason, the employment of molecular biology techniques has been recommended in the guidelines for autopsy investigation of SCD proposed by the Association for European Cardiovascular Pathology [3].

To this aim, 10 ml of EDTA blood and 5 g of myocardium and spleen and/or liver should be taken, frozen, and stored at −80 °C or alternatively stored in RNA later at 4 °C for up to 2 weeks and nucleic acid extraction accomplished through thermocycler.

From fresh tissue, RNA later, autoptic blood in EDTA, or frozen tissue, nucleic acid extraction and gene sequencing can be carried out with success up to 100 % of cases, even when amplicon length is greater than 300 bp. From formalin-fixed and paraffin-embedded tissue (FF-PET), nucleic acid extraction is successful up to 85 % of cases and only when amplicon length is less than 300 bp [4].

A. **Myocarditis.** Lymphocytic myocarditis is the most common form of myocarditis in Western countries, and most of the cases are documented or presumed to be viral in origin. Nonviral infective agents are exceptional and often morphologically distinctive and identifiable by routine histology also including special stains. On the contrary, Classical morphological analysis (histology and immunohistochemistry) has great limits in the detection of viral agents and usually lacks specific cytopathic features, with the rare exception of some forms, like cytomegalovirus (CMV) myocarditis. The development of molecular biological techniques, particularly amplification methods such as polymerase chain reaction (PCR), allows the detection of low copy of viral genomes even from an extremely small amount of tissue such as endomyocardial biopsy. PCR is an enzymatic amplification technique whereby very few copies of RNA or DNA sequences can be amplified more than a millionfold. This allows transformation of a target sequence (i.e., the pathogen in question) from very low numbers to literally millions of copies without cloning technology. The main viruses to be considered when performing molecular pathology studies in the myocardium of patients with a suspicion of myocarditis are adenovirus, CMV, Epstein-Barr virus (EBV), enterovirus, hepatitis C virus, Human Herpes Virus 6 (HHV6), herpes simplex viruses 1 and 2, influenza viruses A and B, and Parvovirus B19 (PVB19). Other infectious agents may be investigated according to the clinical indication (Table 11.1) (Fig. 11.1) [5–7]. However, it has been underlined that the presence of viral genomes does not automatically imply a direct role of viruses in the pathogenesis of myocarditis, since an infective agent detected by PCR/RT-PCR/nested-PCR may be just an innocent bystander. Therefore, it is recommended to use molecular techniques as diagnostic tools ancillary to other mandatory investigations, either clinical or morphological, and apply it with skilled expertise. Positive PCR results obtained on the myocardial samples should always be accompanied by a parallel investigation on blood samples and/or frozen spleen. The absence of a viral genome in the blood and/or spleen sample rules out the possibility of passive blood contamination of the myocardium, while viral blood positivity requires additional investigation by using quantitative PCR analysis. Among the molecular biology techniques used to differentiate viral genomes, gene sequencing allows not only the precise characterization of the infective agent but also can help in assessing the molecular basis of cardiotropism as well as cardiovirulence. Finally, more recently the need of viral genome load quantification has been advanced particularly for some viruses such as PVB19, which are frequently encountered in the diagnostic workup not only of myocarditis but also of healthy transplant donor, of autoptic samples without myocarditis or with borderline myocarditis, and of patients undergoing endomyocardial biopsy for other reasons.

© Springer-Verlag Milan 2016

G. Thiene et al., *Sudden Cardiac Death in the Young and Athletes: Text Atlas of Pathology and Clinical Correlates*, DOI 10.1007/978-88-470-5776-0_11

165

Table 11.1 Suggested PCR primers for viral PCR

Virus	Sequence (5′→3′)	T annealing (°C)	Gene target	Size bp
AV	GCCGCAGTGGTCTTACATGCACATC CAGCACGCCGCGGATGTCAAAGT	65	Exon protein	308
CMV (DNA)	CACCTGTCACCGCTGCTATATTGC CACCACGCAGCGGCCCTTGATGTTT	52	Phosphorylated matrix protein (pp65 e pp71)	399
CMV (RNA)	GTGACCTTGACGGTGGCTTT CGTCATACCCCCCGGAGTAA	57	Early gene	275
EBV	TTCGGGTTGGAACCTCCTTG GTCATCATCATCCGGGTCTC	64	Nuclear antigen 1 (EBNA 1)	268
EV/RV	AAGCACTTCTGTTTCC CATTCAGGGGCCGGAGGA	50	5′ untranslated region (5′-UTR)	297
HCV	GGAACTACTGTCTTCACGCAGA TGCTCATGGTGCACGGTCTA	54	5′ untranslated region (5′-UTR)	255
	GTGCAGCCTCCAGGACCC GGCACTCGCAAGCACCCTAT	56		210
HHV6	GTGAAAACTACGATTCAGGC TTTCGGAACATTGTTGAGC	55	Major DNA-binding protein (U41) gene	264
HSV	CATCACCGACCCGGAGAGGGA GGGCCAGGCGCTTGTTGGTA	60	DNA polymerase	92
INF A	AAGGGCTTTCACCGAAGAGG CCCATTCTCATTACTGCTTC	50	Nonstructural proteins 1 and 2	190
INF B	ATGGCCATCGGATCCTCAAC TGTCAGCTATTATGGAGCTG	57	Nonstructural proteins 1 and 2	241
PVB19	GGTAAGAAAAATACACTGT TTGCCCGCCTAAAATGGCTTT	57	Nonstructural protein 1	218

AV adenovirus, *bp* base pair, *CMV* cytomegalovirus, *EBV* Epstein–Barr virus, *EV/RV* enterovirus/rhinovirus, *HCV* hepatitis C virus, *HSV* herpes simplex virus, *HHV6* human herpesvirus 6, *INF A* influenza A virus, *INF B* influenza B virus, *PVB19* parvovirus B19

B. **Inherited heart diseases.** Overall, 30–40 % of SCD cases in the young are due to genetically, potentially recurrent cardiac disorders, and they include both structural and non-structural heart diseases [1–3]. In these settings, autopsy may represent the first and sole opportunity to make the proper diagnosis, and the tissue sampling at postmortem for genetic testing may be of help, particularly to solve the puzzle of "mors sine materia." As stated in the European guidelines for autopsy investigation of SCD, the final report of a SCD postmortem investigation should always conclude with a clear clinicopathological synthesis (epicrisis) [3].

Although in the majority of SCDs a pathological cause can be identified, the pathologist must also admit that a not negligible proportion of SCD cases present with a structurally normal heart. SCD is considered as occurring in structurally normal heart when a thorough gross, histological, and laboratory examination fails to detect any plausible organic substrate accounting for cardiac arrest ("*mors sine materia*" or sudden unexplained death), after excluding diseases of the coronary arteries, myocardium, valves, great vessels, and conduction system, and unnatural causes of death by toxicological investigation [1]. We believe that the

numbers of SCD with normal heart have been underestimated in the past, due to the overestimation of the so-called borderline findings of uncertain significance (such as fatty infiltration, focal myocarditis, etc.). This fact, together with the nonuniform protocol of investigation adopted until now at autopsy, may explain the great variability in the prevalence of normal heart reported in autopsy studies in the literature. This is well recognized by the scientific community. In fact, the HRS/EHRA/APHRS expert consensus statement on the diagnosis and management of patients with inherited primary arrhythmia syndromes recommends that all victims diagnosed with unexplained SCD syndrome undergo expert cardiac pathology, to rule out the presence of microscopic indicators of structural heart disease before asking for molecular investigation [8]. The vast majority of forensic and general pathologists do not archive tissue in the proper manner. In fact, archived FF-PET is a more easy way of storage and transport and thus is typically the only source of DNA available for procurement. However, DNA from FF-PET is considered error prone and unreliable in comprehensive surveillance of unexplained SCD-associated genes by applying traditional tools of genetic investigation. Thus, the standard autopsy of SD should include archiving "DNA-friendly" material, such as EDTA-preserved blood or frozen tissue (heart, liver, or spleen) to facilitate postmortem genetic testing. More in details, 10 ml of EDTA blood and 5 g of heart and spleen tissues should be either frozen and stored at −80 °C or alternatively stored in RNA later at 4 °C for up to 2 weeks [4].

Nucleic acids are more difficult to extract from FF-PET tissue because of the need to remove the paraffin and to counteract covalent protein–DNA interactions that result from the fixation process. In addition, fixation delay (i.e., perioperative ischemic time), the fixation process, tissue preparation, paraffin embedding, and archival storage contribute to fragmentation, cross-linking, and chemical modification of FF-PET tissue-derived nucleic acids. These changes interfere with many classical molecular analyses requiring high-quality nucleic acids. However, the recent availability of next-generation sequencing (NGS) techniques, with the power to analyze in depth large numbers of short sequences, potentially makes this an ideal technology to apply to the usually fragmented nucleic acids that may be extracted from FF-PET specimens [9, 10]. The development of reliable NGS-based methods for use with low-quality FF-PET tissue-derived nucleic acids would open the diagnostic pathology archives to high-throughput profiling, facilitating extensive retrospective clinical studies. Similarly, the ability to use FF-PET samples for molecular analysis in prospective studies would be of great benefit, by potentially reducing or even eliminating the need for the tedious collection and storage of cryopreserved clinical samples.

This approach should become part of the routine postmortem study of SCD in the young. The message from the dead can save lives. This is particularly true when the heart of SCD victims appears normal at both gross and histological examinations ("*mors sine materia*," SCD with normal heart) [9–15] (Fig 11.2).

In the setting of proven autopsy-negative SCD, comprehensive or targeted (*RyR2, KCNQ1, KCNH2, and SCN5A*) ion channel genetic testing may be considered in attempt to establish probable cause and manner of death and to facilitate the identification of potentially at-risk relatives.

In particular, genetic testing is recommended if circumstantial evidence points toward a clinical diagnosis of LQTS syndrome or CPVT specifically (such as emotional stress or drowning as the trigger of death).

The key question is whether molecular autopsy should be applied to all SCD victims with normal hearts or if it should be used only when clinical evaluation of family members has generated some concern that a genetic cardiac disease might be present. In fact, the advantage of pursuing genetic screening of the unexplained SCD victim over performing clinical evaluation of family members has not been conclusively demonstrated. Last, but not least, the impact of "uncertain results" of genetic testing, represented by the identification of variants that cannot be conclusively defined as "pathogenic," has not been evaluated. In the real world, it has been calculated that 10–15 % of samples from unexplained SCD victims carry a mutation in *KCNQ1, KCNH2,* or *SCN5A*. The addition of the screening of the *RyR2* gene, for mutations that cause CPVT, may increase the yield of molecular autopsy by an additional 5–10 %, thus bringing up to 15–25 %.

At the present time, it seems reasonable to advocate for a combined approach, with parallel clinical assessment of the family members of unexplained SCD victims and molecular autopsy on the proband. This should be based on the need to inform the family of SCD victims that a genetic cause is suspected in the death of their relative, and, therefore, cardiac evaluation is required. At the same time, molecular analysis of the victim's DNA can be performed and the results integrated to increase the accuracy of the diagnosis.

Molecular autopsy results may, in fact, be better interpreted in light of clinical assessment of family members. In case of a "positive" genetic test in the unexplained SCD victims, DNA screening may be extended to family members, to allow the assessment of co-segregation of the mutation with the clinical phenotype and to identify other at-risk individuals (the carriers of the same variant) [16]. As new technologies are reducing the cost of genotyping, it is expected that the prices may rapidly decrease, thus making the postmortem analysis less expensive and more widely used.

11.1   Image Gallery

Fig. 11.1 Molecular pathology of myocarditis in sudden cardiac death Molecular biology techniques identified enterovirus as the main culprit cardiotropic virus. *CMV* cytomegalovirus, *EBV* Epstein Barr virus, *EV* enterovirus, *HSV* Herpes simplex virus, *PVB19* Parvovirus B19

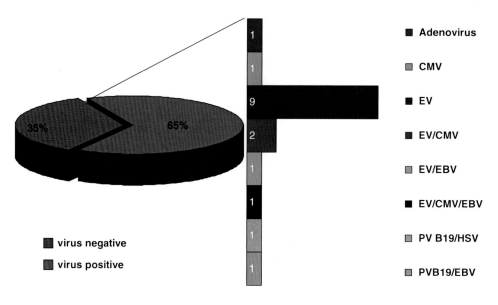

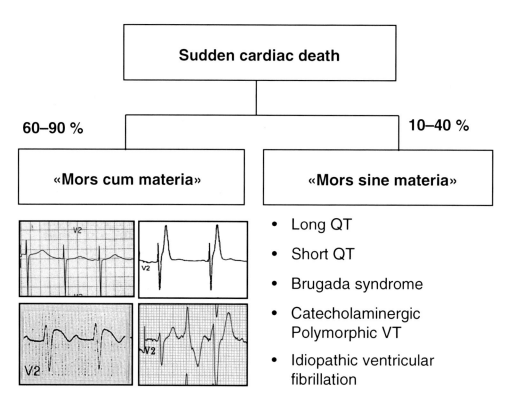

Fig. 11.2 Postmortem genetic testing. Sudden cardiac death shows a substrate ("*mors cum materia*") in 60–90 % of cases and does not show a substrate ("*mors sine materia*") in 10–40 % of cases. The latter consists of long and short QT syndromes, Brugada syndrome, catechol- aminergic polymorphic VT, and idiopathic ventricular fibrillation (still in search of "an author"). In these cases, family screening and post-mortem genetic testing are useful.

References

1. Basso C, Carturan E, Pilichou K, Rizzo S, Corrado D, Thiene G. Sudden cardiac death with normal heart: molecular autopsy. Cardiovasc Pathol. 2010;19:321–5.

2. Thiene G. Sudden cardiac death and cardiovascular pathology: from anatomic theater to double helix. Am J Cardiol. 2014; 114:1930–6.

3. Basso C, Burke M, Fornes P, Gallagher PJ, de Gouveia RH, Sheppard M, Thiene G, van der Wal A. Guidelines for autopsy investigation of sudden cardiac death. Virchows Arch. 2008; 452:11–8.

4. Carturan E, Tester DJ, Brost BC, Basso C, Thiene G, Ackerman MJ. Postmortem genetic testing for conventional autopsy-negative sudden unexplained death: an evaluation of different DNA extraction protocols and the feasibility of mutational analysis from archival paraffin-embedded heart tissue. Am J Clin Pathol. 2008; 129:391–7.

5. Basso C, Calabrese F, Angelini A, Carturan E, Thiene G. Classification and histological, immunohistochemical, and molecular diagnosis of inflammatory myocardial disease. Heart Fail Rev. 2013;18:673–81.

6. Caforio AL, Pankuweit S, Arbustini E, Basso C, Gimeno-Blanes J, Felix SB, Fu M, Heliö T, Heymans S, Jahns R, Klingel K, Linhart A, Maisch B, McKenna W, Mogensen J, Pinto YM, Ristic A, Schultheiss HP, Seggewiss H, Tavazzi L, Thiene G, Yilmaz A, Charron P, Elliott PM. Current state of knowledge on aetiology, diagnosis, management, and therapy of myocarditis: a position statement of the European Society of Cardiology Working Group on Myocardial and Pericardial Diseases. Eur Heart J. 2013;34:2636–48, 2648a–2648d.

7. Leone O, Veinot JP, Angelini A, Baandrup UT, Basso C, Berry G, Bruneval P, Burke M, Butany J, Calabrese F, d'Amati G, Edwards WD, Fallon JT, Fishbein MC, Gallagher PJ, Halushka MK, McManus B, Pucci A, Rodriguez ER, Saffitz JE, Sheppard MN, Steenbergen C, Stone JR, Tan C, Thiene G, van der Wal AC, Winters GL. 2011 consensus statement on endomyocardial biopsy from the Association for European Cardiovascular Pathology and the Society for Cardiovascular Pathology. Cardiovasc Pathol. 2012;21:245–74.

8. Priori SG, Wilde AA, Horie M, Cho Y, Behr ER, Berul C, Blom N, Brugada J, Chiang CE, Huikuri H, Kannankeril P, Krahn A, Leenhardt A, Moss A, Schwartz PJ, Shimizu W, Tomaselli G, Tracy C. Executive summary: HRS/EHRA/APHRS expert consensus statement on the diagnosis and management of patients with inherited primary arrhythmia syndromes. Heart Rhythm. 2013;10: e85–108.

9. Loporcaro CG, Tester DJ, Maleszewski JJ, Kruisselbrink T, Ackerman MJ. Confirmation of cause and manner of death via a comprehensive cardiac autopsy including whole exome next-generation sequencing. Arch Pathol Lab Med. 2014;138:1083–9.

10. Semsarian C, Ingles J, Wilde AA. Sudden cardiac death in the young: the molecular autopsy and a practical approach to surviving relatives. Eur Heart J. 2015;36:1290–6.

11. Hofman N, Tan HL, Alders M, Kolder I, de Haij S, Mannens MM, Lombardi MP, Dit Deprez RH, van Langen I, Wilde AA. Yield of molecular and clinical testing for arrhythmia syndromes: report of 15 years' experience. Circulation. 2013;128:1513–21.

12. Ingles J, Semsarian C. Sudden cardiac death in the young: a clinical genetic approach. Intern Med J. 2007;37:32–7.

13. Tester DJ, Ackerman MJ. The role of molecular autopsy in unexplained sudden cardiac death. Curr Opin Cardiol. 2006;21:166–72.

14. Tester DJ, Medeiros-Domingo A, Will ML, Haglund CM, Ackerman MJ. Cardiac channel molecular autopsy: insights from 173 consecutive cases of autopsy-negative sudden unexplained death referred for postmortem genetic testing. Mayo Clin Proc. 2012;87:524–39.

15. Tester DJ, Ackerman MJ. Postmortem long QT syndrome genetic testing for sudden unexplained death in the young. J Am Coll Cardiol. 2007;49:240–6.

16. Behr E, Wood DA, Wright M, Syrris P, Sheppard MN, Casey A, Davies MJ, McKenna W, Sudden Arrhythmic Death Syndrome Steering Group. Cardiological assessment of first-degree relatives in sudden arrhythmic death syndrome. Lancet. 2003;362:1457–9.

The Northeast Italy, Veneto Region Experience

12

The Veneto Region is located in the Northeast of Italy with Venice as the capital. According to the Italian Census Bureau & Sports Medicine (1979–1999), the overall inhabitants were 437,900 – with the young population (12–35 years) of 1,386,650 and young athletes of 112,790 (M to F=4:1) (Fig. 12.1). In this time interval, the cumulative incidence of SD was 1/100,000/year in young people aged less than 35 years old (SIDS excluded) [1–3]. Among nonathletes, the incidence was 0.9/100,000/year and among athletes was 2.3/100,000/year [1]. Thus the occurrence of SD was 2.5-fold in athletes vs. nonathletes ($p <0.0001$). In the time interval (1980–2013), a total of 650 SCD were studied at postmortem (201 F, 31 %): it was mechanical in 7 % and arrhythmic in 93 % [1] (Fig. 12.2).

Among the mechanical causes, pulmonary embolism accounted for 2 %, aortic rupture for 3 %, and others for 2 %. A congenital or genetic substrate of aortic rupture was always there: Marfan syndrome, bicuspid aortic valve, and aortic isthmic coarctation with or without bicuspid aortic valve. SCD occurred because of hemopericardium with cardiac tamponade, since the aortic dissection with external rupture always involved the intrapericardial ascending aorta (type A).

Coronary atherosclerosis was the cause of SCD in 18 % of cases, usually with a single obstructive atherosclerotic plaque located in proximal descending coronary artery (Fig. 12.3). Acute occlusive thrombosis was present only in 34 % in this group, mostly due to endothelial erosion [4].

In 2 % of cases, the acquired coronary artery disease was coronary dissection, usually in women [5].

Congenital coronary artery abnormalities were the culprit in 5 % of cases, mostly consisting of anomalous origin from the wrong sinus [6].

Myocarditis was diagnosed as the cause of death in 12 %. The inflammatory infiltrate was patchy. Molecular investigation, which was possible to be carried out also in paraffin-embedded myocardium, revealed coxsackievirus as the cardiotropic infective agent in half of the cases [7, 8].

Arrhythmogenic cardiomyopathy resulted to be the third cause accounting for 10 %. The fibrofatty replacement was frequently biventricular and even isolated in the left ventricle or segmental in the right ventricle. The presence of right ventricular aneurysms was a common finding, with the one located in the subtricuspid diaphragmatic region considered a pathognomonic marker of the disease [9, 10].

Hypertrophic cardiomyopathy, with asymmetric subaortic, midventricular, or apical hypertrophy, accounted for 9 %. Severe myocardial disarray and fibrotic scars, located within the asymmetric hypertrophy, were constant findings [11].

Mitral valve prolapse was the only structural disease in 8 % of subjects dying suddenly, largely prevalent in the female gender. In no case death was due to chordal rupture with pulmonary edema. Fibrosis of the papillary muscles and of the posterolateral free wall of the left ventricle was the most likely arrhythmogenic substrate. When available, the ECG disclosed polymorphic premature ventricular beats and repolarization abnormalities in the inferior leads [12].

Conduction system disease, investigated by serial sections technique, was the cause of SCD in 6 %. In the majority, it was an ECG-proven Wolff–Parkinson–White or Lown–Ganong–Levine ventricular preexcitation [13]. In the former, the accessory pathway was detected in the lateral, left or right, AV rings. In the latter, an atrio-hisian bypass bundle ("James" fascicle) or hypoplastic AV node was found at the septal AV junction. There was evidence of atrial myocarditis in half of cases. More rarely, a Lev–Lenegre disease with fibrosis of the branching His bundle was noted, probably explaining cardiac arrest through a sudden AV block.

Dilated cardiomyopathy was the cause of SCD in 4 % of cases. It presented with cardiomegaly with eccentric hypertrophy and biventricular dilatation, in the absence of any other explanation. Histology disclosed cardiomyocyte abnormalities (bizarre nuclei, perinuclear, halo) and patchy fibrosis in keeping with dilated cardiomyopathy [1, 7].

© Springer-Verlag Milan 2016
G. Thiene et al., *Sudden Cardiac Death in the Young and Athletes: Text Atlas of Pathology and Clinical Correlates*,
DOI 10.1007/978-88-470-5776-0_12

Congenital heart diseases were observed in 2 % of cases [14]. They included mostly postoperative tetralogy of Fallot, but also operated subjects for complete transposition by atrial switch. Eisenmenger syndrome along with natural history was also noted in a couple of cases.

Finally, SCD occurred in young subjects in whom the heart appeared normal at gross and histological examination (17 %) [1, 7, 8]. When ECG recordings were available, LQT, SQT, Brugada syndrome, and CPVT were clinically diagnosed. In the absence of ECG, we cannot exclude a concealed Wolff–Parkinson–White syndrome.

Molecular autopsy was employed in the recent years and allowed to reveal pathogenic gene mutations in cases of LQT, Brugada, and CPVT syndromes. Molecular genetic investigation of early cases, "left behind," failed because of the impossibility to extract the DNA from FF-PET (see Chap. 11), confirming that the study should be performed in fresh or frozen preserved tissue [8].

As far as the athletes, arrhythmogenic cardiomyopathy accounted for 23 % of SCD victims, coronary atherosclerosis for 19 %, congenital coronary artery anomalies for 16 %, and hypertrophic cardiomyopathy for only 2 % [1–3, 15]. The discrepancies, when compared with the overall nonathlete population, have to be ascribed to the role played by effort in precipitating SCD [1] (Figs. 12.4 and 12.5). In fact, effort increases five times the risk of SCD in subjects affected by arrhythmogenic cardiomyopathy, because of stretching of the right ventricular free wall. In congenital coronary artery anomalies, the risk ratio between sedentary and sport activity is even higher, i.e. 1:80. By the way, while arrhythmogenic cardiomyopathy discloses subtle ECG abnormalities (T-wave inversion in right precordial leads) [16] (Fig. 12.6) coronary artery disease may exhibit a normal basal and stress ECG, as to escape pre-participation screening even when ECG is employed, like in Italy [3] (Figs. 12.7 and 12.8). On the opposite, the basal ECG is positive in 85 % of hypertrophic cardiomyopathy cases and, as such, allows to raise the suspicion of the disease, which is then confirmed at 2D echocardiography, which is the gold standard for diagnosis and is compulsory in our Country at pre-participation screening in case of doubt [17] (Fig. 12.9). Disqualification from sport activity is lifesaving, and this is the reason why in Italy, the rate of SCD in athletes due to hypertrophic cardiomyopathy is only 2 % vs. 26 % in the United States, a country where the pre-participation screening does not include the use of ECG [18–20]. In the Veneto Region, Northeast of Italy, in the time interval 1979–2004, the annual incidence of SCD declined by 89 % in screened athletes (P for trend <0.001). In contrast, the incidence of SCD did not demonstrate consistent changes over that time in unscreened nonathletes (Fig. 12.10).

12.1   Image Gallery

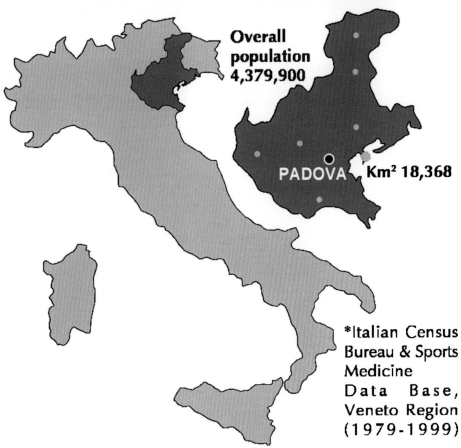

Fig. 12.1 The Veneto Region is located in Northeast Italy with an area of 18,368 km². According to Italian Census Bureau & Sports Medicine database, in the time interval 1979–1999, a mean 4,379,900 overall population was calculated, including 1,386,650 young people and 112,790 young athletes (12–35 years old)

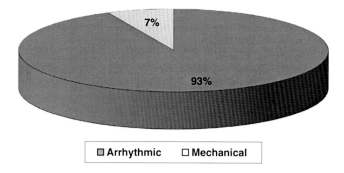

Fig. 12.2 Pathophysiologic mechanisms of sudden cardiac death in young people aged ≤35 years. The majority are arrhythmic in origin (93 %)

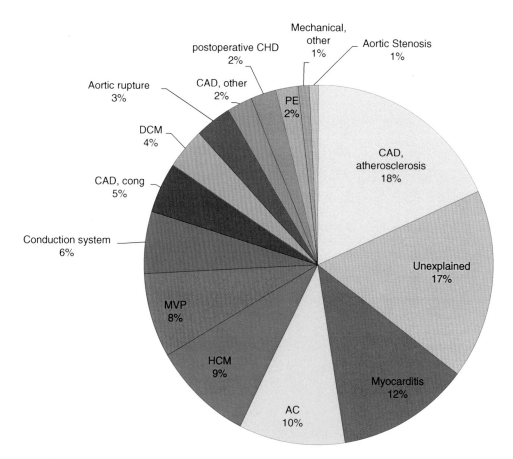

Fig. 12.3 Causes of sudden cardiac death, Veneto Region Northeast Italy, 1980–2013. *AC* arrhythmogenic cardiomyopathy, *CAD* coronary artery disease, *CHD* congenital heart disease, *DCM* dilated cardio-myopathy, *HCM* hypertrophic cardiomyopathy, *MVP* mitral valve prolapse, *PE* pulmonary embolism

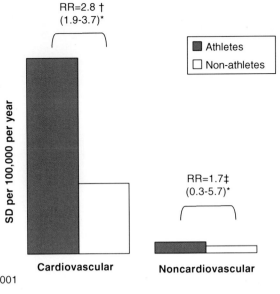

RR=2.8 †
(1.9-3.7)*

RR=1.7‡
(0.3-5.7)*

† p<.00001
‡ p=NS
* 95% CI

Fig. 12.4 Incidence and relative risk (RR) of sudden death (SD) among athletes (*solid columns*) and nonathletes (*open columns*) from cardiovascular and non-cardiovascular causes. Athletes had a 2.8 RR of cardiovascular SD (confidence interval [CI] 1.9–3.7; $p <0.001$), as compared with a 1.7 RR of non-cardiovascular SD (CI 0.3–5.7; $p = 0.39$)

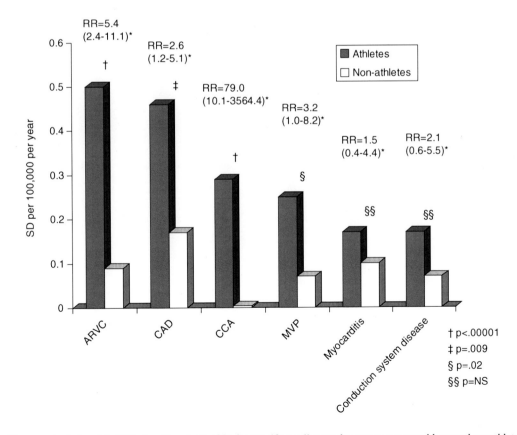

Fig. 12.5 Incidence and relative risk (*RR*) of sudden death (*SD*) for specific cardiovascular causes among athletes and nonathletes. *AC* arrhythmogenic cardiomyopathy, *CAD* coronary artery disease, *CCA* congenital coronary artery anomaly, and *MVP* mitral valve prolapse

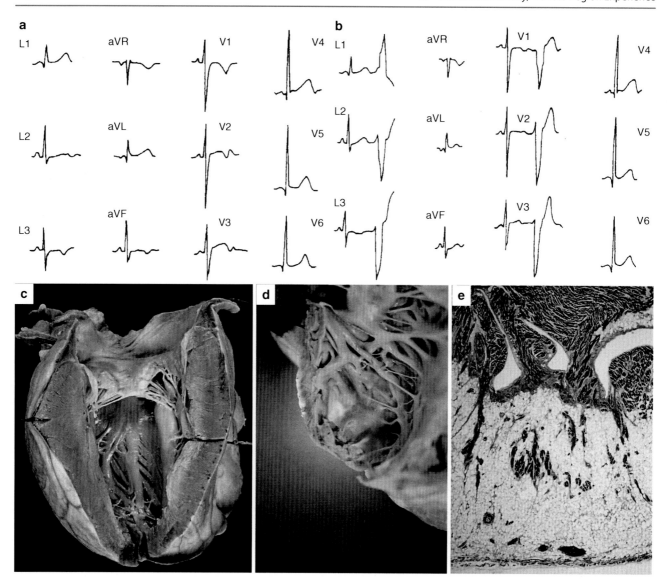

Fig. 12.6 Arrhythmic sudden cardiac death due to arrhythmogenic cardiomyopathy in a 30-year-old competitive athlete during a soccer game (late 1980s, early era of pre-participation screening). (**a**) Note the inverted T waves in the right precordial leads. (**b**) Stress test ECG: a single premature ventricular beat with left bundle branch block morphology. (**c**) At postmortem, the left ventricle was normal. (**d**) The right ventricle had a typical inferior aneurysm. (**e**) At histology, transmural fibrofatty replacement of the right ventricular free wall (Heidenhain trichrome)

Fig. 12.7 Arrhythmic sudden cardiac death due to anomalous coronary artery origin in a 27-year-old rugby player during a game. (**a**) Basal 12-lead ECG with isolated premature ventricular beat (*left*). Effort 12-lead ECG without any sign of myocardial ischemia (*right*). (**b**) View of the aortic root: note the presence of two coronary ostia in the left sinus of Valsalva, with acute angle takeoff of the anomalous right coronary artery (*arrow*)

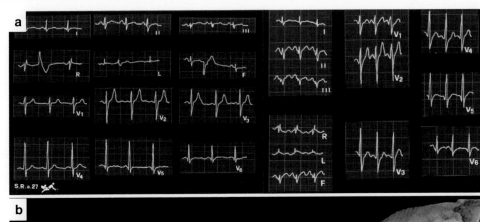

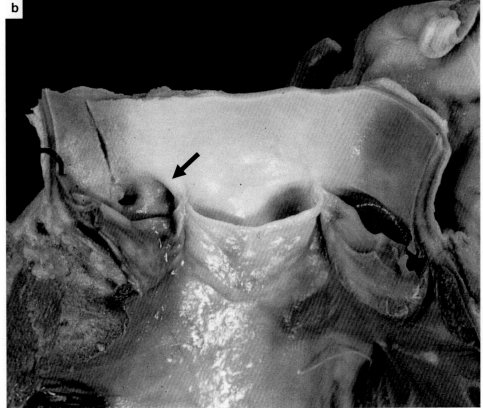

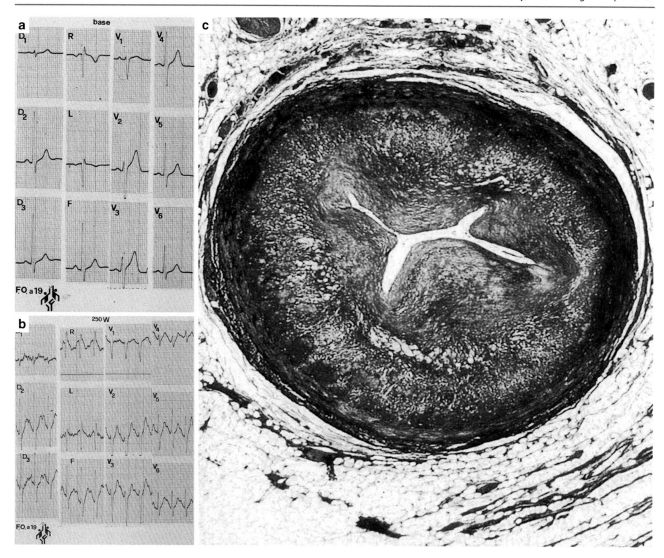

Fig. 12.8 Arrhythmic sudden cardiac death due to coronary atherosclerosis in a 19-year-old basketball player during a game. (**a**) Normal basal 12-lead ECG. (**b**) Effort 12-lead ECG without any sign of myocardial ischemia. (**c**) Histologic section of the proximal left anterior descending coronary artery: note the critical luminal stenosis due to a concentric, mostly fibrocellular, atherosclerotic plaque (Heidenhain trichrome)

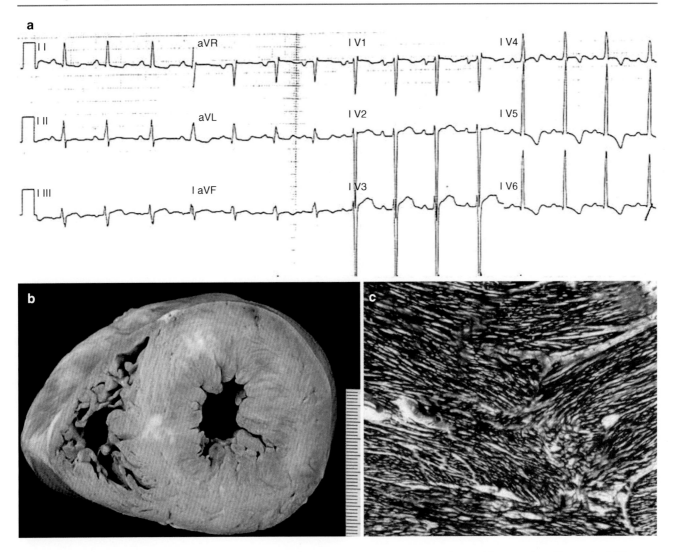

Fig. 12.9 Arrhythmic sudden cardiac death due to hypertrophic cardiomyopathy in a 15-year-old athlete during cycling. (**a**) 12-lead ECG shows deep inverted T waves on V4 to V6. (**b**) Cross section of the heart demonstrates asymmetric septal hypertrophy with grossly visible myocardial scars. (**c**) At histology, extensive fascicular myocardial disarray

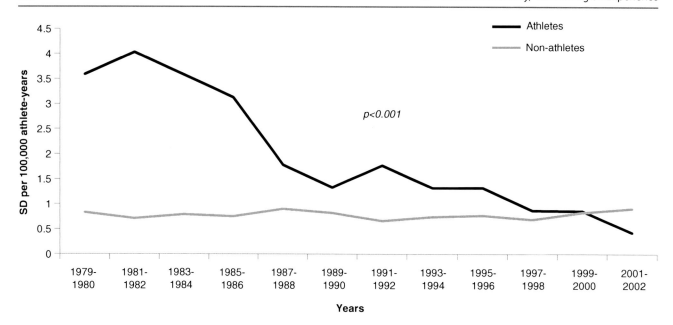

Fig. 12.10 Annual incidence rates of sudden death (SD) per 100,000 person, among screened competitive athletes and unscreened nonathletes 12–35 years of age in the Veneto Region of Italy, from 1979 to 2004. During the study period (the nationwide pre-participation screening program was initiated in 1982), the annual incidence of SD declined by 89 % in screened athletes (P for trend <0.001). In contrast, the incidence of SD did not demonstrate changes over that time in unscreened nonathletes

References

1. Thiene G. Sudden cardiac death and cardiovascular pathology: from anatomic theater to double helix. Am J Cardiol. 2014;114: 1930–6.

2. Corrado D, Basso C, Schiavon M, Thiene G. Screening for hypertrophic cardiomyopathy in young athletes. N Engl J Med. 1998; 339:364–9.

3. Corrado D, Basso C, Pavei A, Michieli P, Schiavon M, Thiene G. Trends in sudden cardiovascular death in young competitive athletes after implementation of a preparticipation screening program. JAMA. 2006;296:1593–601.

4. Corrado D, Basso C, Poletti A, Angelini A, Valente M, Thiene G. Sudden death in the young: is coronary thrombosis the major precipitating factor? Circulation. 1994;90:2315–23.

5. Basso C, Morgagni GL, Thiene G. Spontaneous coronary artery dissection: a neglected cause of acute myocardial ischaemia and sudden death. Heart. 1996;75:451–4.

6. Basso C, Maron BJ, Corrado D, Thiene G. Clinical profile of congenital coronary artery anomalies with origin from the wrong aortic sinus leading to sudden death in young competitive athletes. J Am Coll Cardiol. 2000;35:1493–501.

7. Basso C, Calabrese F, Corrado D, Thiene G. Postmortem diagnosis in sudden cardiac death victims: macroscopic, microscopic and molecular findings. Cardiovasc Res. 2001;50:290–330.

8. Basso C, Carturan E, Pilichou K, Rizzo S, Corrado D, Thiene G. Sudden cardiac death with normal heart: molecular autopsy. Cardiovasc Pathol. 2010;19:321–5.

9. Thiene G, Nava A, Corrado D, Rossi L, Pennelli N. Right ventricular cardiomyopathy and sudden death in young people. N Engl J Med. 1988;318:129–33.

10. Basso C, Thiene G, Corrado D, Angelini A, Nava A, Valente M. Arrhythmogenic right ventricular cardiomyopathy: dysplasia, dystrophy, or myocarditis? Circulation. 1996;94:983–91.

11. Basso C, Thiene G, Corrado D, Buja G, Melacini P, Nava A. Hypertrophic cardiomyopathy and sudden death in the young: pathologic evidence of myocardial ischemia. Hum Pathol. 2000; 31:988–98.

12. Basso C, Perazzolo-Marra M, Rizzo S, De Lazzari M, Giorgi B, Cipriani A, Frigo AC, Rigato I, Migliore F, Pilichou K, Bertaglia E, Cacciavillani L, Bauce B, Corrado D, Thiene G, Iliceto S. Arrhythmic mitral valve prolapse and sudden cardiac death. Circulation. 2015;132:556–66.

13. Basso C, Corrado D, Rossi L, Thiene G. Ventricular preexcitation in children and young adults: atrial myocarditis as a possible trigger of sudden death. Circulation. 2001;103:269–75.

14. Basso C, Frescura C, Corrado D, Muriago M, Angelini A, Daliento L, Thiene G. Congenital heart disease and sudden death in the young. Hum Pathol. 1995;26:1065–72.

15. Corrado D, Basso C, Schiavon M, Pelliccia A, Thiene G. Preparticipation screening of young competitive athletes for prevention of sudden cardiac death. J Am Coll Cardiol. 2008;52: 1981–9.

16. Migliore F, Zorzi A, Michieli P, Perazzolo Marra M, Siciliano M, Rigato I, Bauce B, Basso C, Toazza D, Schiavon M, Iliceto S, Thiene G, Corrado D. Prevalence of cardiomyopathy in Italian asymptomatic children with electrocardiographic T-wave inversion at preparticipation screening. Circulation. 2012;125:529–38.

17. Corrado D, Pelliccia A, Heidbuchel H, Sharma S, Link M, Basso C, Biffi A, Buja G, Delise P, Gussac I, Anastasakis A, Borjesson M, Bjørnstad HH, Carrè F, Deligiannis A, Dugmore D, Fagard R, Hoogsteen J, Mellwig KP, Panhuyzen-Goedkoop N, Solberg E, Vanhees L, Drezner J, Estes 3rd NA, Iliceto S, Maron BJ, Peidro R, Schwartz PJ, Stein R, Thiene G, Zeppilli P, McKenna WJ. Recommendations for interpretation of 12-lead electrocardiogram in the athlete. Eur Heart J. 2010;31:243–59.

18. Maron BJ, Thompson PD, Ackerman MJ, Balady G, Berger S, Cohen D, Dimeff R, Douglas PS, Glover DW, Hutter Jr AM, Krauss MD, Maron MS, Mitten MJ, Roberts WO, Puffer JC. Recommendations and considerations related to preparticipation screening for cardiovascular abnormalities in competitive athletes: 2007 update: a scientific statement from the American Heart Association Council on Nutrition, Physical Activity, and Metabolism: endorsed by the American College of Cardiology Foundation. Circulation. 2007;115:1643–45.

19. Thiene G, Corrado D, Rigato I, Basso C. Why and how to support screening strategies to prevent sudden death in athletes. Cell Tissue Res. 2012;348:315–8.

20. Thiene G, Carturan E, Corrado D, Basso C. Prevention of sudden cardiac death in the young and in athletes: dream or reality? Cardiovasc Pathol. 2010;19:207–17.

Prevention of Sudden Cardiac Death

SCD in the young is usually due to concealed cardiovascular diseases, in the absence of alarming symptoms. The only way to detect and diagnose them in vivo is to submit the apparently healthy young people to a thorough clinical examination, which can unmask the hidden disease [1, 2].

This implies screening of the cardiovascular performance in the young on a large scale. In the past, cardiovascular examination was carried out in male conscripts in Italy, when the military service was obligatory. Since the military service became voluntary and restricted to few people, this opportunity has been lost in our Country. No in-depth visit is carried out at school. The only opportunity, for both males and females, is given by the obligatory pre-participation screening for sport activity eligibility. This is an important occasion not only to identify sick and to ensure healthy people but also to make proper interventions to prevent SCD.

Of course, sport activity is salutary and should be practiced since young age. However, the exercise is a double-edged sword, since it can offer protection in the long term from coronary atherosclerosis in those who are regularly engaged, but can entail in the short term the risk of SCD due to an underlying masked heart disease [3]. SCD can occur during sport activity with 2.5-fold rate than in people not practicing sport and is clearly related to the existence of hidden cardiovascular abnormalities, either structural or functional, of which the subject was unaware [4]. They may involve the aorta, the coronary arteries, the myocardium, the valves, the conduction system, or ion channels. The paradox is that the heart with these concealed morbid entities is compatible with an even excellent performance in terms of cardiac output, but it is vulnerable to sudden electrical instability like ventricular fibrillation or, more rarely, to structural breakdown like aortic rupture.

In the majority of cases, these abnormalities are easily suspected or even diagnosed at basal 12-lead ECG or stress test (see, for instance, cardiomyopathies, ion channel diseases, AV block, preexcitation syndromes). The physical examination alone, as carried out in the US, may skip cardiac diseases at high risk [5], such as hypertrophic cardiomyopathy.

Among 33.735 screened athletes, we were able to detect 22 cases of people affected by hypertrophic cardiomyopathy [6]. Of these 22, 18 (82 %) were suspected thanks to abnormal ECG, whereas only 5 (23 %) had a positive family history or cardiac murmur. Thus, the sensitivity of our system was fourfold that the US one, with obvious implications in terms of SCD prevention [7, 8].

Also arrhythmogenic cardiomyopathy shows ECG abnormalities (large QRS complexes, epsilon waves, inverted T waves in the right precordial leads), which raise the suspicion that there is something wrong. The existence channelopathies is evident at the basal ECG (long and short QT interval, ST segment elevation). The same CPVT syndrome, in which the basal ECG is normal, shows onset of polymorphic ventricular arrhythmias at stress test ECG. Preexcitation syndromes show short PR, with or without delta wave. In all these conditions, the ECG is the only way to identify subjects at risk [8, 9].

Different from the US protocol, which includes only personal and family history with physical examination (not necessarily carried out by physicians) [5], the Italian protocol makes compulsory the employment of the ECG, and if some suspicion arises at the ECG, two-dimensional echo becomes mandatory as well [7, 9]. The last tool is the gold standard for the diagnosis of hypertrophic cardiomyopathy, by detecting left ventricular hypertrophy, either symmetric or asymmetric ($\geq$13 mm).

Figure 13.1 is a flowchart of the protocol of pre-participation screening accomplished in Italy. First level includes family history, physical examination, and 12-lead ECG. If the findings are negative, eligibility for competitive sport is granted. If the findings are positive, a second-level investigation is accomplished, consisting of noninvasive tools (echo, stress test, signal-averaged ECG, Holter monitoring, cardiac magnetic resonance, and angio-computed tomography). If the diagnosis is not yet reached and the doubt persists, a third level of investigation is carried out with the use of invasive tools (coronary angiography, electrophysiologic study, electroanatomic mapping, and even endomyocardial biopsy). In the absence of any cardiovascular disease, green light for eligibility switches on.

© Springer-Verlag Milan 2016

G. Thiene et al., *Sudden Cardiac Death in the Young and Athletes: Text Atlas of Pathology and Clinical Correlates*,

DOI 10.1007/978-88-470-5776-0_13

Disqualification from sport activity is lifesaving "per se." Since the initiation in Italy in 1982 of the nationally wide pre-participation screening (program including ECG), the annual incidence of SCD declined progressively up to 89 % in screened athletes in 2004 (see also Chap. 12) [8].

In contrast, the incidence of SCD did not demonstrate significant changes over the time in unscreened nonathlete young people that had not the opportunity to undergo cardiovascular screening.

Critics argue that false-positive ECG findings may lead to exclusion of many athletes that are not at risk of SD [10, 14, 15]. This is particularly true in certain ethnic groups, like black athletes, with a higher prevalence of ECG abnormalities that are a variant of normal. In our experience, 9 % of 42.386 athletes were found positive at first-level examination, but after further investigation, only 0.2 % were ultimately disqualified [6]. In England, false-positive rates were reported in 3.7 % [14, 15]. Employment of the recently updated guidelines for ECG interpretation has proven to significantly decrease the rate of false-positive among athletes [9]. Certainly, reducing the frequency of unnecessary disqualification and adapting, instead of prohibiting, sport activity (from high static-dynamic to low static-dynamic sports) remains one of the screening objectives.

Coronary artery diseases, either congenital or acquired, may escape detection at ECG. Accelerated coronary atherosclerosis in the young is typically represented by a single plaque in the proximal segment of the left anterior descending artery. It may be totally silent, both in terms of angina and ECG abnormalities at basal 12-lead and stress test recording. A coronary vasospasm, superimposed to the subostructive plaque, has been proven to be a precipitating factor of transient fatal ischemia, something that cannot be reproduced at the pre-participation screening [16]. The relative risk of sport-related SCD in premature coronary atherosclerosis is 2.6, again stressing the role of effort in precipitating cardiac arrest in affected subjects [4].

The relative risk in congenital coronary artery anomalies is even much more (RR = 79.0) as to say that if you are affected by these abnormalities, the risk to die suddenly is only if you make effort [4]. This emphasizes the concept on how much important would be the identification of affected people, because just disqualification from sport activity would be lifesaving. Unfortunately, again, basal 12-lead ECG and stress test ECG appeared normal in cases of coronary artery anomalous origin who died suddenly and thus got eligibility for sport activity [17].

It is clear that in these circumstances, both for acquired and congenital coronary disease, the only way to achieve the diagnosis is the employment of clinical coronary imaging, either noninvasive (computed tomography or cardiac magnetic resonance) or invasive (contrast coronary angiography). Premature coronary atherosclerosis may be suspected on the base of familiarity or lifestyle risk factors (smoke, obesity, hypercholesterolemia, cocaine, and steroid abuse).

There are life-threatening valve diseases (mitral valve prolapse, bicuspid aortic valve), which are electrocardiographi-cally silent and even do not present cardiac murmurs. Mitral valve prolapse is at risk of arrhythmic SCD by ventricular fibrillation (so-called arrhythmic mitral valve syndrome) and bicuspid aortic valve at risk of aortic rupture through aortic dissection. In these circumstances, the only way to get the diagnosis is the use of 2D echo at the time of screening, which to our mind should be added to the first-level investigation.

When a definitive diagnosis of cardiac disease is reached, the sport activity should be restricted or prohibited. Then, the subject becomes a "patient" and as such submitted to well-established therapeutic protocols which concur to prevention of SCD.

Sports disqualification or restriction intervenes on the trigger, whereas drug therapy and ablation point to block the arrhythmic mechanism (Fig. 13.2). Cardioverter defibrillator, whether implantable or automatic external, takes action when cardiac arrest is due to ventricular fibrillation, by delivering electric shock and restoring sinus rhythm (Fig. 13.3). ICD is indicated, according to risk stratification, particularly in subjects with previous aborted sudden death or syncope. The availability of (and expertise of using) automatic external defibrillator should be widespread (sports fields, public places, schools) and become obligatory like fire extinguishers. The latter measure would certainly be of great help in saving the lives of those athletes whose concealed heart defect escaped pre-participation screening, like coronary artery and arrhythmic valve abnormalities.

Sports disqualification, pharmacological or nonpharmacological therapy, and defibrillators are the main measures for SCD prevention. However, although frequently effective measures, these are palliative interventions addressing the arrhythmic symptoms ("symptomatic therapy"). When disease cure will become available through a molecular therapy, by understanding the pathobiological mechanisms underlying the morbid phenomena then the approach to the prevention of SCD in the young will become curative.

Up to 30–40 % of SCD in the young are ascribable to heredofamilial disease (cardiomyopathies, aortic disease, channelopathies, conduction disturbances). Genetic molecular investigation in the affected young is mandatory to establish the causative gene mutation and genome wide investigation is now available, with higher probability to detect the pathogenic defect. Cardiological and genetic screening in first-degree family members is then mandatory to identify even asymptomatic carriers. Considering that SCD may be the first symptom of a cardiac disease in apparently healthy people, the genetic diagnosis in the proband may then be lifesaving for relatives.

Sports pre-participation screening aims not only to identify and disqualify athletes at risk, which is itself a great achievement for SCD prevention. It may save lives of family members by identifying asymptomatic carriers and, last but not least, ensures the remaining 50 % of healthy unaffected people to continue safely a normal life and sport activity/profession, as well as to have children without risk of disease transmission.

13.1   Image Gallery

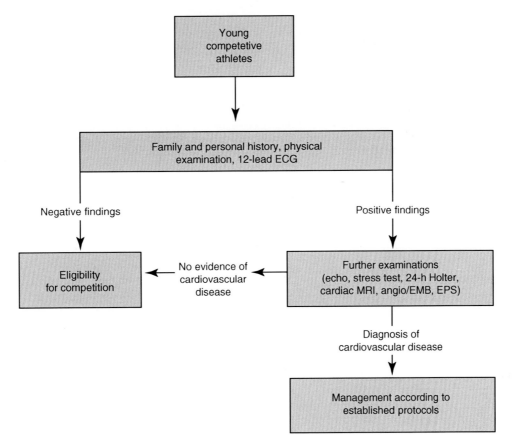

Fig. 13.1 Flowchart of the Italian protocol of pre-participation screening for the prevention of SCD. First-line examination includes family history, physical examination, and 12-lead ECG; additional tests are requested only for subjects who have positive findings at the initial evaluation. Athletes found to be affected by cardiovascular conditions, potentially at risk of sudden death in association with exercise and sport participation, are managed according to the available recommendations for sports eligibility. *Angio/EMB* contrast angiography/endomyocardial biopsy, *EPS* electrophysiologic study with programmed ventricular stimulation, *MRI* magnetic resonance

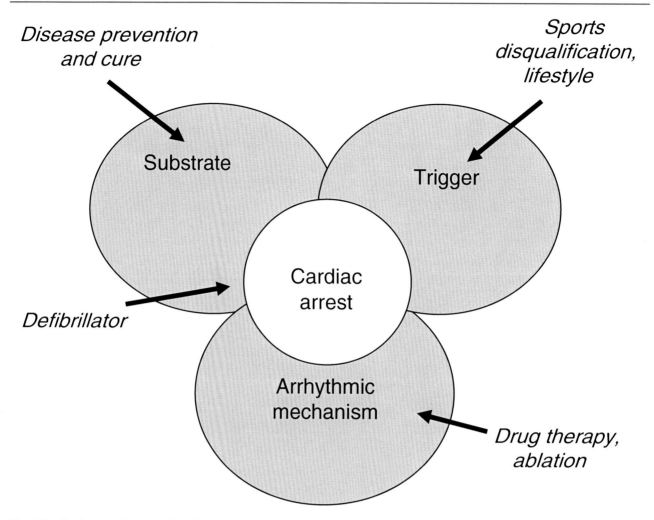

Fig. 13.2 Cardiac arrest is the combination of trigger, substrate, and arrhythmic mechanism. Sport disqualification acts on the trigger; drug therapy and ablation are palliative therapeutic measures. Defibrillator clearly intervenes on the mode of cardiac arrest, namely, ventricular fibrillation. The true prevention and cure should point to block onset and progression of the disease substrate

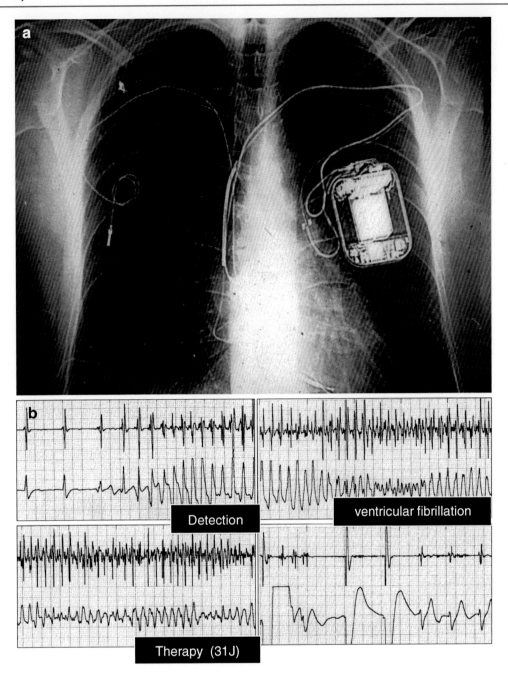

Fig. 13.3 Chest radiogram of a patient with arrhythmogenic cardiomyopathy and recurrent episodes of cardiac arrest. A cardioverter defibrillator was implanted (**a**) to prevent sudden death with lifesaving interruption of ventricular fibrillation (**b**)

References

1. Thiene G. Sudden cardiac death and cardiovascular pathology: from anatomic theater to double helix. Am J Cardiol. 2014;114:1930–6.
2. Thiene G, Carturan E, Corrado D, Basso C. Prevention of sudden cardiac death in the young and in athletes: dream or reality? Cardiovasc Pathol. 2010;19:207–17.
3. Maron BJ. Sudden death in young athletes. N Engl J Med. 2003;349:1064–75.
4. Corrado D, Basso C, Rizzoli G, Schiavon M, Thiene G. Does sports activity enhance the risk of sudden death in adolescents and young adults? J Am Coll Cardiol. 2003;42:1959–63.
5. Maron BJ, Thompson PD, Ackerman MJ, Balady G, Berger S, Cohen D, Dimeff R, Douglas PS, Glover DW, Hutter Jr AM, Krauss MD, Maron MS, Mitten MJ, Roberts WO, Puffer JC. Recommendations and considerations related to preparticipation screening for cardiovascular abnormalities in competitive athletes: 2007 update: a scientific statement from the American Heart Association Council on Nutrition, Physical Activity, and Metabolism: endorsed by the American College of Cardiology Foundation. Circulation. 2007;115:1643–455.
6. Corrado D, Basso C, Schiavon M, Thiene G. Screening for hypertrophic cardiomyopathy in young athletes. N Engl J Med. 1998;339:364–9.
7. Decree of the Italian Ministry of Health, February 18, 1982. Norme per la tutela sanitaria dell'attività sportiva agonistica (rules concerning the medical protection of athletic activity). Gazzetta Ufficiale 5 Mar 1982. p. 63.
8. Corrado D, Basso C, Pavei A, Michieli P, Schiavon M, Thiene G. Trends in sudden cardiovascular death in young competitive athletes after implementation of a preparticipation screening program. JAMA. 2006;296:1593–601.
9. Corrado D, Pelliccia A, Heidbuchel H, Sharma S, Link M, Basso C, Biffi A, Buja G, Delise P, Gussac I, Anastasakis A, Borjesson M, Bjørnstad HH, Carrè F, Deligiannis A, Dugmore D, Fagard R, Hoogsteen J, Mellwig KP, Panhuyzen-Goedkoop N, Solberg E, Vanhees L, Drezner J, Estes 3rd NA, Iliceto S, Maron BJ, Peidro R, Schwartz PJ, Stein R, Thiene G, Zeppilli P, McKenna WJ. Recommendations for interpretation of 12-lead electrocardiogram in the athlete. Eur Heart J. 2010;31:243–59.
10. Maron BJ, Haas TS, Doerer JJ, Thompson PD, Hodges JS. Comparison of U.S. and Italian experiences with sudden cardiac deaths in young competitive athletes and implications for preparticipation screening strategies. Am J Cardiol. 2009;104:276–80.
11. Corrado D, Pelliccia A, Bjørnstad HH, Vanhees L, Biffi A, Borjesson M, Panhuyzen-Goedkoop N, Deligiannis A, Solberg E, Dugmore D, Mellwig KP, Assanelli D, Delise P, van-Buuren F, Anastasakis A, Heidbuchel H, Hoffmann E, Fagard R, Priori SG, Basso C, Arbustini E, Blomstrom-Lundqvist C, McKenna WJ, Thiene G, Cardiovascular pre-participation screening of young competitive athletes for prevention of sudden death: proposal for a common European protocol. Consensus Statement of the Study Group of Sport Cardiology of the Working Group of Cardiac Rehabilitation and Exercise Physiology and the Working Group of Myocardial and Pericardial Diseases of the European Society of Cardiology. Eur Heart J. 2005;26:516–24.
12. Thiene G, Corrado D, Schiavon M, Basso C. Screening of competitive athletes to prevent sudden death: implement programmes now. Heart. 2013;99:304–6.
13. Thiene G, Corrado D, Rigato I, Basso C. Why and how to support screening strategies to prevent sudden death in athletes. Cell Tissue Res. 2012;348:315–8.
14. Maron BJ, Friedman RA, Caplan A. Ethics of pre-participation cardiovascular screening for athletes. Nat Rev Cardiol. 2015;12:375–8.
15. Basavarajaiah S, Boraita A, Whyte G. Ethnic differences in left ventricular remodeling in highly-trained athletes: relevance to differentiating physiologic left ventricular hypertrophy from hypertrophic cardiomyopathy. J Am Coll Cardiol. 2008;51:2256–62.
16. Corrado D, Basso C, Poletti A, Angelini A, Valente M, Thiene G. Sudden death in the young. Is acute coronary thrombosis the major precipitating factor? Circulation. 1994;90:2315–23.
17. Basso C, Maron BJ, Corrado D, Thiene G. Clinical profile of congenital coronary artery anomalies with origin from the wrong aortic sinus leading to sudden death in young competitive athletes. J Am Coll Cardiol. 2000;35:1493–501.

Index

A
Adrenal haemorrhage, 5, 17
Anabolic androgenic steroids, 98, 106, 107
Anomalous pathway, 123, 129, 130
Aortic aneurysm, atherosclerotic, 5, 14
Aortic dissection, 5, 14, 23, 109, 113–117, 171, 184
Aortic valve stenosis, 74, 109–112
Asthma, 4, 9, 150
Asystole, 4, 5, 123, 141
Atherosclerotic plaque
  erosion, 21, 36, 42, 171
  fibro-atheromatous, 27, 33, 42
  fibrocellular, 21, 36, 42, 178
  rupture, 4, 21, 23, 33, 35, 42, 152, 171
Athlete heart, 74, 152
Atrio-ventricular block, 5, 123–124, 131, 141, 143, 152, 171, 183

B
Berry aneurysm, 4, 8
Bicuspid aortic valve, 5, 109, 111–115, 137, 171, 184
Bioprosthesis, 5, 16
Brechenmacher fascicle, 123
Brugada syndrome, 124, 132, 143, 144, 168, 172

C
Cardiac magnetic resonance, 23, 74, 110, 183, 184
Cardiac rupture, 5, 152
Cardiac tamponade, 5, 11, 23, 109, 113–117, 151, 153, 174
Cardiac tumors, 124
Cardiomyopathy
  arrhythmogenic, 1, 2, 73–75, 86–94, 143, 152, 171, 172, 174–176, 183, 187
  dilated, 1, 22, 74, 98, 107, 171, 174
  hypertrophic, 1, 24, 73–74, 76–85, 152, 171, 172, 174, 179, 183
Catecholaminergic polymorphic ventricular tachycardia, 143, 144, 146, 167, 168, 172, 183
Celothelioma of the atrioventricular node. See Cystic tumor of the atrioventricular node
Cerebral hemorrhage, 4, 150
Channelopathies. See Ion channel disease
Chlamydia pneumonia, 97
Cocaine, 21, 23, 36, 42, 44, 98, 184
Complete transposition of the great arteries, 137
Coronary artery
  arteritis, 22, 23
  congenital anomalies, 3, 6, 22–24, 137, 151, 171, 172, 175, 184
  dissection, 23, 50–54, 171
  embolism, 21, 22, 40, 46, 151
  high take-off, 24, 67, 152
  origin from the opposite wrong sinus, 23, 24, 58, 59, 137, 171

origin from the pulmonary trunk, 23, 57, 152
  origin of the left circumflex from the right, 151, 152
Coronary
  thrombosis, 4, 21–23, 28, 32–40, 42, 48, 151, 152, 158, 171
  vasospasm, 21–23, 184
Corrected transposition of the great arteries, 137, 141
Cystic tumor of the atrioventricular node, 124, 133, 152

D
Defibrillator
  automatic external 5, 184
  implantable cardioverter, 2, 4, 149, 184, 187
  jacket, 97
Dissecting aneurysm. See Aortic dissection
Double-outlet right ventricle, 137
Duodenal ulcer, 5

E
Early repolarization, 143
Ebstein's anomaly, 110, 121
Echocardiography, 23, 172, 183, 184
Eisenmenger syndrome, 137, 138, 152, 172
Electrocardiography, ECG, 1, 2, 5, 21, 24, 41, 73, 74, 89, 119, 123, 125, 126, 128, 129, 131, 132, 143–145, 149–152, 163, 171, 172, 176–179, 183–185
Electro anatomic mapping, 74, 183
Endomyocardial biopsy, 74, 97, 165, 183, 185

F
Epilepsy, 4, 149
Fibroma, cardiac, 124

G
Gastric ulcer, 5
Genetic testing, 166–168
Giant cell arteritis, 22

H
Hemopericardium, 5, 11–13, 109, 152, 171
Histocytoid cardiomyopathy. See Purkinje cell tumor
Hypoplastic AV node, 123, 128, 171

I
Idiopathic infantile cardiomyopathy. See Purkinje cell tumor
Idiopathic left ventricular hypertrophy, 74, 152
Ion channel disease, 1, 5, 22, 75, 97, 124, 143, 144, 167, 183

© Springer-Verlag Milan 2016
G. Thiene et al., *Sudden Cardiac Death in the Young and Athletes: Text Atlas of Pathology and Clinical Correlates,*
DOI 10.1007/978-88-470-5776-0

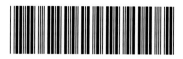